THE CHALLENGES OF MEDICAL PRACTICE
VARIATIONS

2014

610

ECONOMIC ISSUES IN HEALTH CARE

General editors

Professor Gavin Mooney
Institute of Social Medicine
University of Copenhagen
2200 Copenhagen N, Denmark

Dr Alistair McGuire
Centre for of Socio-Legal Studies,
and Pembroke College
University of Oxford
Oxford OX2 6UD, England

THE CHALLENGES OF MEDICAL PRACTICE VARIATIONS

Edited by

Tavs Folmer Andersen

and

Gavin Mooney

Institute of Social Medicine
University of Copenhagen, Denmark

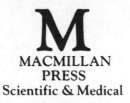

MACMILLAN
PRESS
Scientific & Medical

First published 1990

Published by
THE MACMILLAN PRESS LTD
Houndmills, Basingstoke, Hampshire RG21 2XS
and London
Companies and representatives
throughout the world

Filmset by
Wearside Tradespools, Fulwell, Sunderland

Printed in Hong Kong

British Library Cataloguing in Publication Data
The challenges of medical practice variations.
1. Medicine. Decision making. International aspects
I. Andersen, T. Folmer (Tavs Folmer)   II. Mooney,
Gavin, 1943–   III. Series
610
ISBN 0–333–47508–9
ISBN 0–333–47509–7 pbk

Contents

Preface

The objective of *The Challenges of Medical Practice Variations* is to stimulate debate about the research and policy implications of the variations in medical practices from various perspectives, including efficiency, equity and effectiveness, but also health policy, health service management, clinical practice and the role of the medical profession. The focus is international but, in particular, European.

The book has been a genuinely joint process not only by the editors, but also by all the contributors. That is wholly appropriate, as it is our view that the challenge of medical practice variation does not only lie with the medical profession, nor only with medical research: variation involves many facets and many disciplines and professions.

The publication of this book, which is the first dealing solely with the topic of medical practice variation, is also the joint product of the efforts of the staff and board of the CCC – the Copenhagen Collaborating Center for the Study of Regional Variations in Health Care. To all of them, past and present, we owe a special debt.

The process involved in preparing the book may be worth mentioning. As editors we drew up a series of outlines for the contributions we sought and then got the agreement of the authors we had selected to write them. We wrote the introductory chapter and circulated this to all the contributors. They submitted synopses of their chapters, on which we commented, and then wrote their chapters which again we commented on before this final product emerged.

Finally, we should like to thank Maria Kapitzke and Annelise Nielsen for their secretarial assistance in the preparation of manuscripts.

Copenhagen, May 1989   T.F.A.
                                                                                        G.M.

The Contributors

Tavs Folmer Andersen
Copenhagen Collaborating Center
Institute of Social Medicine
University of Copenhagen
Panum Institute
Blegdamsvej 3
2200 Copenhagen N
Denmark

Gwyn Bevan
Department of Community Medicine
St. Thomas's Hospital
London SE1 7EH
England

Ruth Brazauskas
Department of Business Administration
Faculty of Management
University of Manitoba
Winnipeg, Manitoba R3T 2N2
Canada

Marsha M Cohen
Department of Community Health Sciences
Faculty of Medicine
University of Manitoba
Winnipeg, Manitoba R3T 2N2
Canada

Robert G Evans
Department of Economics
University of British Columbia
400-2194 Health Sciences Mall
Vancouver, B.C. V6T 1Z6
Canada

Jonathan Lomas
Department of Clinical Epidemiology and Biostatistics
Faculty of Medicine
McMaster University
Hamilton, Ontario L8S 4M4
Canada

Alistair McGuire
Centre for Socio-Legal Studies, and Pembroke College
University of Oxford
Oxford OX2 6UD
England

Klim McPherson
Department of Community Medicine
Oxford University
Gibson Labs Radcliffe Infirmary
Oxford OX2 6HE
England

Gavin Mooney
Institute of Social Medicine
University of Copenhagen
Panum Institute
Blegdamsvej 3
2200 Copenhagen N
Denmark

Albert G Mulley, Jr.
General Internal Medicine
Massachusetts General Hospital
Fruit Street
Boston, MA 02114
USA

Leslie L Roos
Department of Business Administration
Faculty of Management
University of Manitoba
Winnipeg, Manitoba R3T 2N2
Canada

Sandra M Sharp
Department of Business Administration
Faculty of Management
University of Manitoba
Winnipeg, Manitoba R3T 2N2
Canada

Frede Vestergaard
Berlingske Weekendnews
G1. Mønt 1
1147 Copenhagen K
Denmark

John E Wennberg
Department of Community and Family Medicine
Dartmouth Medical School
Hanover, NH 03755
USA

CHAPTER 1

Medical Practice Variations: Where Are We?

Tavs Folmer Andersen and Gavin Mooney

WHY IS PRACTICE VARIATION BECOMING A CHALLENGE?

The existence of variations in modern medical practice has become a challenge for all health care systems in the industrialised world. To meet this challenge, major revisions have to be undertaken concerning many common practices in modern medicine. Practice variation may be seen primarily as a symptom, but it is a symptom which reveals the presence of a very fundamental syndrome, deeply rooted in all highly developed health care systems, a syndrome which will require radical therapy sooner or later.

Why should the mere existence of variation in modern medical practice be thought to provide a sufficiently powerful force to incite a minor revolution in the basis of the health care sector and in our understanding of modern medical practice? Variation is an intrinsic feature of most human practices. Most everyday activities in modern industrialised societies do not, in general, conform to homogeneous patterns across time and space. However, there are certain aspects which for historical reasons make the health care sector appear to stand out as steadfast and true: rock-solid in the torrent of uncertainties that represent modern life.

Medical practice – in contrast to most other social practices – has the image of being based on solid, scientific grounds. We have all been brought up with an understanding that medical care was established through a continual process of interaction between medical practice and medical science, with ever more sophisticated knowledge becoming available to the defenders of our precious health, the medical profession. The development of present-day medical sciences has taken place in a very explicitly international context, which has contributed substantially to the image of modern health care as being based on a unified body of comprehensive scientific knowledge.

The perception of modern medical practice as a coherent scientifically based activity has, by and large, been accompanied by a general fascination by the technologically advanced level of new innovations.

1

The place to be is on the technological frontier. The introduction of ever more complicated therapeutic interventions has created a picture of the medical profession as being in command of healing powers, unintelligible to people outside the medical profession. A monopoly of medical knowledge and power has thus emerged, and the lay population has increasingly found itself in a highly dependent role, having to seek advice from that unified brotherhood of medical agents, who are at the same time executing the treatment of choice.

There is little doubt that the treating physician often has to act as the patient's informing and guiding agent in the pursuit of what is best for the patient. Physicians are not just suppliers but also demanders in health care. However, there has to be some doubt about the merits of this unified brotherhood acting not only on behalf of individual patients, but also on behalf of the societies they claim to serve.

What is the nature of this 'issue of variation', which may turn out to have the necessary power to challenge such well-established realities and myths about medical care and the medical profession?

A new combination of disciplines in health services research is beginning to provide powerful methods, which first of all draw attention to the existence of enormous differences from one place to another in the way that current medical practice is conducted. Second, they provide a starting point for understanding potential causes of these variations, one cause being, for example, the lack of an adequate scientific basis for many common medical interventions. Third, they allow us to identify specific areas in common medical practice where such uncertainties imply significant variations in health outcomes and utilisation of resources. Finally, this combination of disciplines in health services research provides an opportunity to fill in the gaps in our current knowledge through an emerging strategy for non-experimental assessment of health care.

As a result of this concerted research activity, a new picture of modern medical practice is emerging. It is becoming evident that, whereas in advanced health care systems medical practice at large has been considered a coherent unified activity, highly significant variations in treatment methods seem to be the rule rather than the exception in modern medical care.

The scientific basis of many prevailing medical interventions is to a large extent inadequately developed, and many common treatments have been launched without ever having been subjected to thorough scientific evaluation.

The medical profession has to cope with clinical decision making in an environment of wide ranges of uncertainty. What may – seen from one perspective – appear to be a unified brotherhood turns out to be diversified into a wide variety of subgroups with highly different practice styles for reasons that, while remaining somewhat obscure, appear not to be explicative in medically scientific terms.

A more or less mythological image of medical care as a professionally homogeneous, scientifically based activity is giving way to a more realistic, but far more challenging, actuality of variability and uncertainty. We shall all have to cope with this 'new reality' of medical care and the possible change of climate that it involves. The medical profession will have to deal in an explicit way with decision making under clearly 'less-than-certain' circumstances, but at the same time meet the responsibility of systematically filling out the gaps in current knowledge about effectiveness of alternative treatments. The administrators of health services and health policy makers will have to acknowledge the uncertainties that are associated with a large proportion of common medical practices and, without advocating simplistic and often insufficient containment solutions, challenge the decision makers to pursue efficient practice styles. The people that are served by the health services will have to realise that their physicians are not in command of perfect knowledge about the best way to treat their health problems, but will also themselves have to accept a greater share of responsibility in decision making under uncertainty.

In summary, the development of health services research is gradually providing more and more visible evidence about the details of health services utilisation. Providers, consumers and administrators are becoming more knowledgeable as a result. The visibility allows a greater appreciation of the major contributions of modern health care to the maintenance of healthy populations but, at the same time, it reveals all the weaknesses and inadequacies. This is one major reason why variations in medical practice are becoming a challenge in our time.

WHAT EXACTLY IS MEANT BY VARIATION IN MEDICAL PRACTICE?

Many people are aware of individual propensities among health professionals to prefer specific types of treatment to others, and the concept of variation in medical practice is not a new one. However, when we deal with practice variation in the current context, it is important to stress the quantitative aspects – and the need for accurate information about health care activities – that is, the occurrence of activities seen in relation to the size of the population being served. This epidemiological perspective has a long history, and early studies of regional variations in hospital admissions provided important information for the battle against fatal contagious diseases of the nineteenth century. In the modern context of health care epidemiology, quantitative studies of variations in medical practice can be traced back to the 1930s (Glover, 1938). However, a fully fledged strategy of investigation required the installation of large-scale administrative databases as well as modern computing facilities (Wennberg and Gittelsohn, 1973).

The increasing availability of such health care utilisation databases in a number of countries has made it possible to produce precise estimates of population-based rates of utilisation and to compare the average rates of individual countries as well as the rates of small areas within each country. Databases are now available in many countries which permit very detailed analyses of activities based on diagnostic and therapeutic information for small geographic areas. It is, for example, possible in many countries to estimate the age-specific rates of surgical removal of the uterus for specific indications, such as fibroids and menstrual disorder, among inhabitants of small geographic areas such as municipalities, towns or postal code areas. When properly aggregated into larger 'market areas', most of these are predominantly served by one single hospital or other service point such as a clinic, and the population-based rates will thus provide evidence on the activity of that particular hospital. Using this methodology, studies of variation in medical practice have now been performed in many health care systems for many activities all over the world (CCC Bibliography, 1985, 1987).

HOW MUCH DOES MEDICAL PRACTICE ACTUALLY VARY?

Practice variation may be studied at many different levels ranging from the individual clinical decision makers to the level of entire health care systems.

International comparisons of patterns of utilisation in health care systems with high technical standards were performed in the 1960s. It became evident from these studies that, despite the fact that the health professionals in all the health care systems basically shared the same body of scientific knowledge as a basis for their activities, huge differences in practice were occurring. For a large number of diseases and treatments the population-based rates of admission were consistently very high in the USA compared with the UK (Pearson et al., 1968). For some diseases Sweden followed similar patterns of admission to those observed in the USA, whereas for some treatments the rates were even lower than those in the UK. With regard to specific surgical operations, it was found that the number of operations with similar rates of utilisation in the three health care systems was very limited – for example, inguinal herniography and operations for peptic ulcer. Most operations occurred at very different rates in the three countries – for example, tonsillectomy and adenoidectomy, for which the rates varied by a factor of 2–4.

Other comparisons of the USA, Canada and England and Wales from the 1960s found similar differences between the patterns of utilisation of surgical operations. The highest and lowest frequencies of surgery differed by a factor of 2 (Bunker, 1970), but low variation was observed for some procedures, such as appendectomy, while the frequency of some procedures, such as cholecystectomy and tonsillectomy, was more than five times higher in Canada than in England (Vayda, 1973).

Seen in the light of the common scientific basis of clinical decision making in each of these countries, such differences in utilisation are striking. However, it is important to note that each health care system is adjusting its activities to a specific social, historical and cultural setting, in which many different factors may influence the performance and fundamental objectives of the health care systems. A striking feature is presented in figures showing that the rates of compulsory admissions to psychiatric institutions in Scandinavia varied substantially in 1982. For Sweden they were 248 per 100 000, for Norway 109 and for Denmark 26 (Høyer, 1985). It is relevant to add that if one asked any Scandinavian about the rank ordering of these numbers, even if they knew nothing of psychiatry, they would, given existing knowledge of the three countries, almost certainly guess right.

Turning from the macro level of cross-national comparisons to the micro level of small geographical areas within individual countries, the pattern of practice variation proves to be even more striking. In principle it would be attractive, if one were able to define geographical regions around each treatment facility in such a way that the inhabitant population, when treated, would all go to the same clinic. However, this is rarely possible, because referral of patients tends to cross geographical boundaries in a way that prevents a simple and clear picture from emerging.

A very useful methodology for approximating the ideal situation has been developed, and has been named the method of 'small area variation studies' (Wennberg and Gittelsohn, 1973). The starting point for defining these 'small areas' or 'market areas' is the smallest administrative geographical unit which is available in the data at hand. Each of these is then attached to one particular treatment unit, with responsibility for the majority of interventions (admissions or treatments) that occur among the inhabitant population. After attaching all micro areas to treatment units, all areas belonging to the same unit are lumped together into one 'market area', which is predominantly (but not entirely) served by that particular unit. Estimated population-based rates of intervention for such market areas provide useful information on the activity of the corresponding treatment unit. The rates of intervention are rarely entirely attributable to one 'responsible' hospital, because a minor proportion of interventions in the area tend to be performed by other hospitals. However, in most situations the approximation is sufficiently good to allow inference about clinical decision making in the corresponding treatment units. Studies of variations in clinical practice with larger geographical units, such as counties or regions, tend to conceal variations that may be clinically as well as statistically significant. For example, the rate of hysterectomy in one county of Denmark was estimated to be close to the national average, while market areas within that county showed variations by a factor of 5–6 (Andersen *et al.*, 1987).

Access to administrative databases and modern computing facilities have made such investigations easy to perform in many health care systems, and the literature on small-area variations in medical practice is constantly growing (CCC Bibliography, 1985, 1987).

WHAT ARE SOME OF THE TYPICAL PATTERNS OF UTILISATION THAT EMERGE FROM SMALL-AREA VARIATION STUDIES AROUND THE WORLD?

Many studies have been devoted to surgical interventions, for which the quality of data tends to be relatively high compared with diagnostic information and information about other medical treatments. A relatively consistent pattern of variations seems to emerge from studies of different health care systems. Some procedures tend to be associated with a high degree of variability in rates of utilisation within each health care system, while other procedures appear to be consistently characterised by low variation. Comparison of small-area variation for seven surgical procedures was carried out for areas in the USA, the UK and Norway (McPherson *et al.*, 1982). It was consistently found that tonsillectomy rates showed the largest amount of variation *within* each country, with rates of the high areas 3–5 times the rates of the low areas. The average rate in the data for the USA was about twice the average for the UK, which again was about twice the Norwegian rate. Despite these differences in the surgical levels *between* each country, the internal amount of variation seemed to be stable across the three health care systems. Procedures such as appendectomy and hernia repair showed consistently low levels of variation within the three health care systems, while cholecystectomy, prostatectomy, hysterectomy and haemorrhoidectomy were characterised by an intermediate level of variations. The authors concluded:

'... for most of the procedures we examined, a specific pattern of variation exists across international boundaries, and is independent of the national method of organising or financing medical care. Furthermore, procedure-specific variation occurs in countries, where prevailing rates of use are considerably lower than in the United States' [p. 1313].

These results have spurred an increased interest in more extensive international comparative studies of variations in medical practice, taking advantage of the administrative databases which have become available in many countries.

Although – as previously mentioned – the majority of small-area variation studies have thus far been concerned with surgical procedures, some have also studied the entire range of hospital-based medical activities. In a study from New England all non-obstetric medical and surgical hospital admissions were included and classified on the basis of so-called diagnosis-related groupings (Wennberg *et al.*, 1984). In line with results from earlier studies, it was found that hysterectomy showed a pattern of variation with high rates about four times the low rates. While this range of variation may appear to be fairly wide, the study revealed a striking pattern for other activities. The vast majority (85%) of all the classified hospital-based diagnoses and activities turned out to vary more between small areas than did hysterectomy. Among the categories with a very high degree of variation were adult bronchitis and asthma, kidney and urinary tract infections, hypertension, peptic ulcer, paediatric pneumonia, knee operations, D.&C. and tonsillectomy. None of the medical causes of admission was characterised by low variation, while hernia repair and hip repair (except joint replacement) varied a little.

Returning, then, to our initial question about the extent to which modern medical practice is a variable enterprise, there is a firm empirical basis for a preliminary conclusion which flies in the face of many prevailing ideas about medical practice being a unified coherent activity across the industrialised world. Substantial and even gross variations occur between countries as well as between small geographical areas within countries. Substantial variations in utilisation of modern medical care seem to be more of an overwhelming rule than an exceptional phenomenon. Practice variation has revealed to a greater extent than ever before, and in a way which denies the essentialism of modern medicine, that medical practice floats on a sea of uncertainty.

THE CHALLENGES

It is now established that substantial variations in various forms of

medical practice exist both across different countries and across different small areas within individual countries. Out of that statement arise
many challenges. Here we wish to deal with these under two broad
headings: What are the challenges? Who has the responsibility for
responding to them?

What Are the Challenges of Medical Practice Variation?

However, before going further, we need to stress that the task is not to
eliminate variations. Some variations are 'legitimate': for example, those
arising because of different background morbidity. Others may be
legitimate, depending on the ethos and ideology of the society or
community in which they are based: rural and urban populations may
value health and health services differently. Yet other variations may be
deemed 'illegitimate': for example, those arising because some individual clinicians are not aware of existing knowledge on outcomes.
Others still, which arise because knowledge of outcomes is not available
to the profession, may have to be accepted in the short run, even if in the
longer run they might also be considered illegitimate. It is these
illegitimate variations in both the short and long run which are of most
concern in what follows.

Let us take a step back for a moment and consider what we believe to
be fairly firm ground. Clinicians do different things when treating what
appear to be comparable patients. There are various ways to make
treatment decisions and many different factors that might enter the
clinician's decision-making paradigm. Possible factors, whatever the
process, include:

(1) The doctor's judgement of the possible outcomes, both beneficial
and adverse.

(2) The doctor's judgement of the probabilities of these outcomes.

(3) The utilities attached to these outcomes by the doctor and/or the
patient.

(4) The attitude to risk of the doctor and/or the patient.

(5) The degree of paternalism of the doctor/desire for autonomy on
the part of the patient in the decision-making process, including their
willingness to give and receive information.

(6) The availability of facilities and their costs at the hospital level
(beds, doctor time, etc.), but perhaps also at the primary care/
community level, including the patient's family resources.

(7) The nature of the clinician's reward system, where reward can
relate to any factor which provides any form of incentive or disincentive
on the clinician's behaviour.

This is a rather imposing list. Yet we would not claim that it is necessarily complete. What it does serve to show is how potentially difficult clinical decision making can be and the problems involved for the clinician in acting as the patient's agent.

It is not our intention to attempt to sort out what factors matter more and what less – beyond highlighting one major consideration. Whatever the explanation for variations, there is a general agreement that they would be much less in a world of certainty. It is the presence of uncertainty in clinical decision making that allows variations to blossom. However, beyond that various theories, sometimes competing, sometimes complementary, present: professional uncertainty, particularly about outcomes, allowing for practice style variations (see, for example, Wennberg *et al.*, 1982); supplier-induced demand (Evans, 1974), which argues that doctors can shift the demand curve outwards, thereby 'inducing' demand; the closely related agency relationship, which suggests that the doctor acts as an agent for the ill-informed patient (Arrow, 1963); Roemer's law, which states that a built bed is a filled bed (Roemer and Shain, 1959); the concept of need, which, while there is little agreement on its definition, is normally seen as being dominated by the clinician acting in the patient's interest (Williams, 1978); and so on. All of these in some way or other relate to uncertainty and the lack of information on the part of the consumer leading to the situation where the supplier (doctor) dominates the health care market.

Many observers have commented on how the nature of the commodity health care leads to this supplier domination. Perhaps the following quotation from Weisbrod (1978) best summarises the position:

> 'What a buyer wants to know is the difference between his state of well-being with and without the commodity being considered. For ordinary goods, the buyer has little difficulty in evaluating the counter-factual – that is, what the situation will be, if the good is not obtained. Not so for the bulk of health care (and legal representation, to cite another example). The noteworthy point is not simply that it is difficult for the consumer to judge quality before the purchase (as it also is in the used car case), but that it is difficult even after the purchase.'

There is even uncertainty over the terminology. Wennberg *et al.* (1982) emphasise physician or professional uncertainty about the outcomes of the treatments and the probabilities of the outcomes (but also include uncertainty regarding the involvement of the patient in the decision-making process and whether it is the patient's utilities and attitudes to risk that are allowed to count). Among economists a distinction is often drawn between ignorance, uncertainty and risk. All of these terms involve consideration of possible future states of the world, each with some chance of occurring. 'Ignorance' covers those where the decision maker knows neither the states of the world nor the probabilities of their occurrence; with 'uncertainty', the states of the world are known but not the probabilities; and, finally, 'risk' is used for those situations where both the states of the world and the probabilities are known.

It is important to note here that even when there is agreement between clinicians about the possible outcomes and the probabilities, i.e. the assessment of *risk* is the same, it is still possible for there to be no consensus about the benefit of treatment. This can occur because the utility assessment of the outcomes is different or because the attitude to risk of the decision makers differs, i.e. one may be more risk-averse than another. Patients may also vary in respect of their willingness to receive (and ability to digest) information about their health status, treatment and prognosis and in respect of their desire to retain some elements of consumer sovereignty in the decision-making process. Such factors may also lead to variations in treatment strategy, but these can nonetheless be conducive to maximisation of patient benefit.

However, we would not question the importance attached by Wennberg *et al.* (1980) to improvement of our knowledge about outcomes. In many ways, it is puzzling that the outcomes of so many common procedures are subject to so much 'professional uncertainty' – particularly so, given the involvement of so many countries in clinical trials.

The difficulties here are great, and there are several reasons for them. Most fundamentally there is a historical legacy of practices becoming common without having been sufficiently evaluated in scientific trials. Further, the process of measuring health outcomes is itself problematical (for a good review of the issues, see Culyer, 1983). Establishing precisely what the objectives of a particular procedure are is sometimes a source of disagreement. Setting up good studies to measure both short- and long-term effects is difficult, time-consuming, costly and sometimes unethical. Given the pace of technological innovation, results of such studies can be out of date even before they are published. There may be a lack of other incentives to conduct these effectiveness studies. Trying to incorporate all utility-bearing aspects – not just health outcomes but also information and the decision-making role of the patient – is seldom even attempted.

Perhaps the most important study needed in this area of effectiveness analysis is a study to investigate the reasons that so few studies are done, which genuinely result in reducing professional uncertainty. Why are these aspects of evaluation not an integral part of both medical practice *per se* and health care policy?

It is difficult – most would argue impossible – to conduct efficiency studies without first having done or incorporating effectiveness studies.

However, it is perhaps being too puristic to see matters in these terms. At a time when there is considerable concern – and it is unlikely to go away in the immediate future, if at all – about the ability of the wealth of nations to cope with the demands or needs for health care, there is at least an incentive to look at medical practice variations in resource terms. Faced with the clinicians' all-too-frequent lack of convincing evidence on health outcomes on the basis of which they might otherwise justify their use of society's scarce resources, politicians may well want to emphasise cheapness rather than efficiency. And while we wait for the effectiveness studies to be conducted, the pressure to improve efficiency does not abate. Decisions regarding efficiency are and will continue to be made on the basis of inadeqate effectiveness information. How best to cope in these circumstances has to be a matter of considerable concern, at least in the short run, but perhaps the push for efficiency can be one of the major incentive mechanisms at the level of health services to improve knowledge of effectiveness. In other words, if the doctors cannot show better than they have to date that $2x$, $3x$ or $5x$ is better than x, is it surprising that cost-cutting politicians will prefer x?

Whatever the evidence on the implications of practice variation for effectiveness and efficiency, the very existence of such variations is an indication of geographical inequities. Individual patients in different geographical areas are being treated differently for reasons that appear unfair or unreasonable. While one can debate precisely what is meant by equity in health care and can wonder about how important it is to gain equality of access to potentially ineffective treatment, nonetheless the existence of medical practice variations does provide in our view *prima facie* evidence of inequities.

Many research inquiries (see, for example, Illsley and Svensson, 1986) have examined and monitored variations across different areas and groups in society in terms of health status and health care utilisation to indicate the presence of inequalities. Fewer have done so in terms of variations in access – and fewer still in terms of variations in access to common standards of care. Medical practice variations provide an added incentive for a closer examination of the meaning and desirability of equity in health care.

This is particularly so in the context of regional resource allocation formulae such as 'RAWP' in the United Kingdom (Department of Health and Social Services, 1976). Attempting to allocate resources equitably to different regions may well be desirable, but stopping there may not be enough if the different regions then use a substantially different mix of practices.

Where Lies the Responsibility for Responding to the Challenges?

Something is wrong. Unless that message is accepted by medical doctors, health care policy makers and the population when they view the accumulated evidence on medical practice variations, then little will change. And change is needed.

Perhaps the most fundamental issue is that of attempting to ensure that in the future, at least more so than in the past, 'best medical practice' is pursued. Given the gross variations that do exist and accepting that some proportion of the variations is legitimate, it is still difficult to agree that all procedures at all levels can be judged to be 'best'.

Planning of health services and the evaluation of different patterns of resource deployment need to take account of medical practice variations and, more fundamentally, need better knowledge of effectiveness. In the interest of reducing 'illegitimate' variations, policy makers need to adopt methods of resource allocation, particularly budgeting systems, which will provide the right set of checks and balances on clinician behaviour. It may even be that changes in financing and remuneration systems need to be examined in terms of their effectiveness in ameliorating the adverse effects of variations. Essentially the message to the policy makers is that they need to look beyond the provision of health care and accept a greater responsibility for the systematic and routine *evaluation* of health care.

A more fundamental issue still which policy makers must address is that of informing the community served by the health service. It is not clear that the public is yet ready to face the fact of the uncertainty and variation in medical practice that exists. Of course there is something reassuring for the patient in believing that the doctor (a) is only interested in the patient's well-being and (b) does so with knowledge and certainty. In so far as the facts are different, it behoves policy makers to inform the public of this.

The responsibility that rests on the medical profession in the face of the evidence on practice variations is both great and grave. The basis of medical science is not what was thought.

Discussing the (false) basis on which modern medicine has been based, Juul Jensen (1987) highlights two principles: that of 'essentialism', i.e. 'that there is a fixed "natural" border between disease and health'; and 'the principle of specific treatment which states that having revealed a disease, the doctor can, at least in principle, find the one correct treatment'. It has now to be accepted that these two principles are dead. Uncertainty is the current reality. The goal for the future is not to return to the principles of essentialism and of specific treatment. What is now needed is to accept that different outcomes are possible from a treatment and that these *and* the probabilities of their occurrence can be established.

Clinicians must be encouraged, cajoled, given incentives, perhaps finally forced to look more closely at their practices and examine more explicitly the basis on which they make their decisions. Formalised decision analysis and medical decision science are slowly becoming more accepted within the profession. The recently formed European Society for Medical Decision Making follows in the steps of its US counterpart in attempting to promote studies using such systematic approaches. Yet such analyses are far from being pervasive. They are still looked upon with suspicion by many clinicians.

More, better-designed clinical trials which genuinely attempt to link meaningful output measures to the clearly specified objectives of the procedures are needed. Health status measurement in such trials needs more often to grapple with what matters to patients' welfare – quality of life in all its dimensions – rather than simply settling for some neat and measurable end-point such as death.

More fundamentally, medical practice variations point to the necessity for changes in medical education. There is a need to undertake some major reorganisation of the medical curriculum to allow the realities of the evidence on practice variations to become a driving force in the training of future doctors. It would be unreasonable to suggest that decision making based on biological criteria be supplanted totally, but to supplement it with more psychological reasoning, combining probability theory with risk assessment, and utility theory in decision making models is now necessary. Doctors need some basic training in economic thinking. They need to be exposed to social sciences more generally and to population-based health sciences. However, how to promote such change is problematical. It is urgently needed.

Health services researchers also carry some responsibility to meet the challenges of medical practice variations, but it is at a rather different level. It is they who have provided the knowledge of the existence of the variations. It is their evidence that is cited in the first part of this chapter.

Where their responsibility lies is in furthering the descriptive studies; improving outcome measurement; testing different hypotheses to explain the variations; questioning conventional theories; experimenting with different incentive mechanisms to promote effective and efficient health care; and moving health services and medical practice more in the direction of evaluation and audit.

If the health services and the medical profession do accept the responsibilities we have indicated, then this will inevitably place considerable demands on the health services research community. It is our belief that three particular facets of the work of that community then need to change. First, health services research is variable in quantity, quality and status across different countries. There is an urgent need for international collaboration and cross-fertilisation. Second, in the specific context of the concerns of this chapter there are three, at present largely separate, research disciplines that need to become more closely integrated: health services epidemiology; medical decision making; and health economics. Third, researchers need more often to move out of their ivory towers and learn the language and the problems of the health policy makers and the medical doctors

Then the prospects of integrating research with evaluation in both medicine and health care will be more readily realised.

CONCLUSION

The challenges of medical practice variation are real. The existence of such variations has to be a source of concern in modern-day health care and may even become a cause for alarm. But, given a recognition of the need to grapple with the variations and the causes that lie behind them, the real challenge here is to create a better basis for both modern medicine and health care. It is to the specifics of this challenge that the following chapters are devoted.

REFERENCES

Andersen, T. F., Madsen, M. and Loft, A. (1987). Regionale variationer i anvendelsen af hysterektomi. *Ugeskrift for Lager*, **36**, 149, 2415–9

Arrow, K. J. (1963). Uncertainty and the welfare economics of health care. *American Economic Review*, **53**, 941–73

Bunker, P. (1970). Surgical manpower. A comparison of operations and surgeons in the United States and in England and Wales. *New England Journal of Medicine*, **282**, 3, 135–44

CCC Bibliography on Regional Variations in Health Care (1985, 1987). Institute of Social Medicine, Copenhagen

Culyer, A. J. (1983). *Health Indicators*. Martin Robertson, Oxford

Department of Health and Social Services (1976). *Sharing Resources for Health in England: Report of the Resource Allocation Working Party*. HMSO, London (The 'RAWP' Report)

Evans, R. G. (1974). Supplier-induced demand: some empirical evidence and implications. In Perlman, M. (Ed.), *The Economics of Health and Medical Care*. Macmillan, London

Glover, J. A. (1938). The incidence of tonsillectomy in school children. *Proceedings of the Royal Society of Medicine*, **31**, 1219–36

Høyer, G. (1985). Tvangsinnleggelser og tvangsretensjon i psykiatriske institusjoner – en sammenligning av regelverk og praksis i de skandinaviske land. *Nordisk Psykiatrisk Tidsskrift*, **39**, 147–57

Illsley, R. and Svensson, P. G. (1986). *The Health Burden of Social Inequities.* WHO, Copenhagen

Juul Jensen, U. (1987). *Practice and Progress. A Theory for the Modern Health Care System.* Blackwell, Oxford

McPherson, K., Wennberg, J. E., Hovind, D. B. and Clifford, P. (1982). Small-area variations in the use of common surgical procedures: An international comparison of New England, England, and Norway. *New England Journal of Medicine*, **307**, 21, 1310–14

Pearson, R. J. C., Smedby, B., Berfenstam, R., Logan, R. F., Burgess, A. M. and Peterson, O. L. (1968). Hospital caseloads in Liverpool, New England and Uppsala. An international comparison. *The Lancet*, September 7, 559–66

Roemer, R. and Shain, M. (1959). Hospital costs relate to the supply of beds. *The Modern Hospital*, **92**, 71–3

Vayda, E. (1973). A comparison of surgical rates in Canada and in England and Wales. *New England Journal of Medicine*, **289**, 1224–9

Weisbrod, B. A. (1978). Comment on M. V. Pauly. In Greenberg, W. (Ed.), *Competition in the Health Care Sector*, Proceedings of a conference sponsored by the Bureau of Economics. Aspen Systems, Germanstown

Wennberg, J. E., Barnes, B. A. and Zubkoff, M. (1982). Professional uncertainty and the problem of supplier-induced demand. *Social Science and Medicine*, **16**, 811–24

Wennberg, J. E., Bunker, J. P. and Barnes, B. (1980). The need for assessing the outcome of common medical practices. *Annual Review of Public Health*, **1**, 277–95

Wennberg, J. E. and Gittelsohn, A. (1973). Small area variations in health care delivery. A population-based health information system can guide planning and regulatory decision-making. *Science, New York*, **182**, 1102–7

Wennberg, J. E., McPherson, K. and Caper, P. (1984). Will payment based on diagnosis-related groups control hospital costs? *New England Journal of Medicine*, **311**, 5, 295–300

Williams, A. (1978). Need – an economic exegesis. In Culyer, A. J. and Wright, K. G. (Eds.), *Economic Aspects of Health Services.* Martin Robertson, Oxford

CHAPTER 2

Why Do Variations Occur?

Klim McPherson

INTRODUCTION

The previous chapter has set the scene for discussing variation. This chapter will establish a set of yardsticks with which we can observe and compare variation. In medical practice an observer might gain the impression that one health professional will be more inclined to do one thing while another might prefer an alternative treatment. Such an observation will, in general, be difficult to interpret, simply because each medical encounter and each decision is unique and it will rarely be clear that the situations being compared are strictly comparable. Is the disease the same? Is the severity the same? Do the patients have similar expectations? Do the patients have similar desires? What about other exogenous constraints on the decision, such as the queue of patients outside the door, the availability of hospital provision or of drugs? And, of course, different professionals are trained by different people and they learn their craft by different experiences. Moreover, certain decisions may be rewarded differently from others, depending on the system of health care delivery.

The existence of variation in medical practice should not be surprising and it is not difficult to postulate plausible reasons to explain such variation. The challenge of medical practice variation lies in our ability to measure and understand such variation and to be reasonably secure in assigning causation. If we can measure and compare the extent of practice variation and understand its causes, we can then proceed to measure and understand its consequences so that not only will we know that there is variation (or that there is not), but also we may understand better what the expected losses and benefits associated with each decision may be.

The main substantive finding of the study of variation is that for many diagnoses there appears to be quite enormous uncertainty concerning the appropriate method of treatment. As we shall see, arriving at the above conclusion requires a great deal of assiduous analysis, which uncovers a degree of implied uncertainty in clinical decision making which many people find disconcerting. The extent of this uncertainty sometimes allows a variety of ethical clinical decisions which would never be remotely tolerated by any ethical committee considering a randomised clinical trial in which patients were to be allocated at random to the two extremes of current treatment practice, in order to evaluate relative efficacy (Cochrane, 1972).

By the same token, there are many treatments for which there is scarcely any variation apparent between populations and which, as we shall discuss, therefore provide evidence for the existence of a consensus about the appropriate treatment. It is vital to recognise that the study of variation is as useful in recognising implied certainty as uncertainty. Where this consensus, when it exists, can be related to a coherent body of evidence, then use rates between populations can be taken as a measure of appropriateness. There is currently a tendency in some health service circles to regard utilisation rates, *per se*, as an index of appropriateness (Goldacre and Griffin, 1983). Quite often high rates are regarded as an index of high productivity and therefore to be encouraged! Thus, the primary purpose of the analysis of variation is to identify areas of important uncertainty and to distinguish them from areas of relative certainty. This is particularly necessary in medicine, for the overt, and perhaps gratuitous, declaration of uncertainty can be disconcerting and therefore counter-effective.

Herein lies an essential paradox in the study of medical practice which is uniquely illuminated by the dispassionate study of variation. Medicine is widely held to be a science, but many medical decisions do not rely on a strong scientific foundation, simply because such a foundation has yet to be fully explored and developed. Hence, what often happens in the decision-making process is a complicated interaction of scientific evidence, patient desire, doctor preferences and all sorts of exogenous influences, some of which may be quite irrelevant. This tends to happen under the overall umbrella of science, for two reasons. The first is that patients who are concerned with their symptoms are happier if they can believe that what is being done can be justified scientifically. But the second has to do with the professional aspirations of health professionals, who can command more respect if what they do can be seen to require professional expertise. This, of course, means that a further challenge to the study of medical practice variation is that it is sometimes intrinsically threatening to the perceived role of medicine. For to find evidence of uncertainty where none was thought to exist by the experts can be undermining to a legitimate authority.

UNITS OF MEASUREMENT

As we have mentioned, the first requirement of the study of practice variation is the ability to measure it. We need, therefore, a measure which has known characteristics and uses. How can we know where there is practice variation and where there is not? We certainly cannot take large numbers of sample patients to many clinical situations to find out whether the decisions taken were or were not homogeneous. In fact, this has been done on one or two occasions but cannot be used routinely. Where it has been done, it tends to illuminate the problem which we shall discuss in detail below. A classic example was the study of children with acute and recurrent tonsillitis who were referred to one ENT specialist for an opinion about surgical treatment (American Child Health Association, 1934). His recommendation was that half would benefit from tonsillectomy but the other half would not. When the second half were referred again to another ENT specialist, his recommendation was that half would benefit from tonsillectomy but the other half would not. This process was repeated and on each repetition the aggregate decision was the same. However, the poor children participating in the study must have wished for better medical care. However, the important question is which of these bewildering choices would have constituted the better care?

There are other examples, both anecdotal and systematic, which illustrate the existence of practice variation at an individual level. Such examples are important and fascinating in understanding the general phenomenon. However, the purpose of this chapter is to develop the rudiments of a theory of analysis and exposition with a view to understanding the causes of variation. In the above example the causes of such variation must be, at the very least, professional uncertainty about who will benefit from surgery. In fact, the observation is compatible with something approaching total uncertainty, in which the clinical decision is completely random and owes nothing to science, or even to professional experience. But such methods of measurement are only exceptionally available. Moreover, tonsillectomy is much studied and known to be one of the most discretionary, and therefore variable, of medical or surgical recommendations (Bloor and Venters, 1978). As such, it can be used as a yardstick for testing the following methodology.

The first and most simple step is to use population-based rates for particular medical or surgical procedures. Thus, one knows the population for which such rates might apply in an epidemiological sense, the age and sex and prevailing illness patterns will be understood to some degree, and the availability of health services for such populations will be known. Thus, in any year the rate of cholecystectomy in a population may be 250 per 100 000. Such a rate may be the consequence of many thousands of decisions taken on many thousands of patients over the course of that year, and therefore clearly measures something to do with medical decisions. On the other hand, it does not necessarily provide insight into any individual clinical decisions. But the problem with observing individual decisions is that it is never clear that they are entirely comparable, with respect to the nature or severity of the illness or the preferences of the patient. Thus, population-based rates have characteristics similar to those of any average measure.

If, for instance, in a different population the cholecystectomy rate was 400 per 100 000 population, then there could be many plausible explanations for such a difference. But there remains little doubt that, for one reason or another, this latter population undergoes cholecystectomy at a higher rate that the first population. The important point now is to isolate the reason (or reasons) for this, because only then will such a comparison become useful. It is helpful, at this stage, to enumerate the possible reasons for observing different population-based rates in medical practice. Once we have an exhaustive list, it will become easier to consider and identify plausible reasons for variation in particular cases.

REASONS FOR DIFFERENCES IN RATES

Morbidity

The populations being compared may have different prevailing rates of illness for which the index intervention is appropriate. Thus, perhaps for dietary reasons or genetic reasons, the rate of development of gallstones in the first population is lower than in the second. Clearly, if true, such an explanation could alone cause the observed difference in rates. In general, morbidity rates are difficult to measure, because mostly they will be measured by admission rates or consultation rates and could therefore be confounded with practice variations themselves. In essence, this represents one of the most intractable problems in the interpretation of differences in rates. Of course, genuine surveys of morbidity could give insights into differences in rates, but such things are expensive to do reliably.

Demography

The two populations may have very different age and sex characteristics. In this example gallbladder disease is known to be more common among females than among males and is more common as one gets older. If, then, the second population consisted of a higher proportion of elderly females, then, similarly, this could explain the observed difference. Hence, all such comparisons should be standardised for the age and sex distribution of the populations. In this way any residual differences will be unlikely to be a consequence of different demography.

Random

Any rate is essentially calculated by dividing the number of events by the population at risk. Thus, in small populations the number of events may be few and, consequently, a rate may vary from one year to the next, or from one population to the next, in a random manner which may have very little to do with aggregate clinical decisions or population characteristics. Thus, care has to be taken when comparing rates that the differences are not attributable merely to chance fluctuations.

Availability of Resources or Supply

This category consists of the many exogenous influences on medical decisions which have to do with the supply of resources – that is, bed availability, manpower levels, availability of operating theatres or anaesthetists, waiting list, and so on. Such factors will inevitably affect clinical decisions. They will do so either by effectively prohibiting a particular decision because the necessary resources are not available at the right time or, more subtly, by imposing some rationing which ensures that priorities (informal or formal) are set for the use of these resources. For example, in the first population considered above, relative shortage of general surgeons will ensure that only the most acute or dangerous gallstones will be treated immediately by surgery. Often when there are severe constraints, patients may be advised to alter their diet and thus may completely avoid surgery. By the same token, as facilities or manpower expand, such patients may increasingly be offered surgery, in extremes as a preventive measure – a prudent (?) insurance against acute cholecystitis occurring in inconvenient places or at inconvenient times (Fitzpatrick *et al.*, 1977). Also, in constrained health systems patients may be discouraged from attending at all if they suspect that a wait is involved, or a scruffy, full waiting-room.

Almost all extremes of health-care supply are observed where in some countries, with annual health budgets of a few pounds per head, almost nothing is provided to the majority of the population, to others where average expenditure might be several hundred pounds, but among some sections of the community health resources are consumed at a far higher rate (Maxwell, 1981; OECD, 1987). Usually, in the latter situation these populations are wealthy and the provision of health care facilities has assumed a high priority over many years. Such facilities will be used in preference to leaving them idle and, accordingly, patients with 'appropriate' needs will often be forthcoming.

Included in this general category, although not strictly a measure of the availability of resources, will be the method of reimbursement for medical services. Fee-for-service systems tend to provide high levels of availability for acute services for patients with adequate medical insurance and low levels for patients without such cover – in particular, for chronic care. On the other hand, prepayment systems provide an incentive to underprovide to minimise expenditure. In general, for these reasons, method of reimbursement is hopelessly confounded with both availability and, of course, clinical judgement (see below). As George Bernard Shaw (1906) has eloquently pointed out, to give clinicians a financial reward for one decision and none for another should give rise to an expectation of as much impartiality as from judges who might be paid according to the quantity of their innocent (or guilty) verdicts! In the face of genuine uncertainty, exogenous and irrelevant considerations are bound to come to the fore.

Clinical Judgement

As has been indicated, some clinicians may have different opinions about the relative merits of various treatment options for a given condition. They may also differ in their diagnoses. They may have been taught differently or their reading of the literature may simply indicate those preferences or their own personal experience may suggest that some things work better or more safely than others. Moreover, their interpretation of the evidence may put a lot of weight on their particular expertise. Thus, if they consider themselves to be good at some things and not so good at others, then such matters will affect their judgement. In particular, if, for instance, an episode of treatment goes badly wrong at some time, then such an experience could colour attitudes considerably.

Note that none of these considerations need necessarily lead to the right conclusion, in the methodological sense of being unbiased. Thus, in medicine there are many opportunities for deception in the interpretation of evidence, made in an uncontrolled manner and inevitably on relatively few patients. Nonetheless, it remains possible for such evidence to appear utterly convincing, which is not to say that any beliefs are necessarily wrong, merely that they can be. When clouded with financial and professional implications, such beliefs are, of course, more difficult to test. Herein lies the uncertainty.

We are here concerned with the nature of the evidence a well-informed clinician has at his or her disposal. When the word 'uncertainty' is used, it can have a pejorative implication which implies that the uncertainty is attributable to ignorance or laziness. This may be so, but is not the concern here. The determination of the efficacy, in all its dimensions of outcome, is often extremely difficult. Hence, 'to be uncertain' is here used to mean that the consequence of doing one rather than another intervention in a given disease state is very imprecisely understood by everyone.

Patient Expectation or Demand

Clearly, different patients have different desires and expectations related to their symptoms. At the most basic, some hesitate before consulting medical opinion, while others see a doctor with the slightest symptoms. Given a particular condition, some patients prefer an interventionist approach, while others expect the opposite. Balancing perceived benefits and risks against each other is accomplished in totally different ways by different people. In the end it is these considerations which should determine the rate of any medical intervention, given a known incidence of morbidity of a community. With certain diagnosis and complete information on the outcome associated with all possible interventions, then all that is left are patient preferences for particular outcomes, conditioned by public policy on expenditure and priorities, both social and economic. If all observed variations were a manifestation of no more than such informed consumer choices, then they would present few challenges.

Prevailing Custom

Possibly independent of supply, there might be a separate component which determines the rate of intervention. Some communities might eschew certain kinds of medical intervention more than others notwithstanding availability or recommendation. Such things might affect the dominant case-mix of admission procedures. In essence, this is a conditioning of either prevailing medical opinion or patients' preferences by long-standing custom or tradition (Aaron and Schwartz, 1984).

Rates for Previous Years for Organ Removal

Given high rates of intervention for particular operations in previous years, the rates for current periods may be affected by consequent organ loss. Thus, population estimates do not provide the proper denominator for the calculation of rates. For example, in some parts of America the rate of hysterectomy is, between the ages of 45 and 65, more than 1% per annum. That means that for these twenty years alone the cumulative risk is more than 18%. Hence, rates of hysterectomy among 65-year-old women will underestimate considerably the true risk for women with wombs. Thus, to compare the rates between communities requires relatively low rates in previous years for those procedures which can only be done once, or the rates ought to be related to the estimated population at risk (Gittelsohn and Wennberg, 1976).

Omissions from Data Sources

Increasingly, in the UK, for example, hospital use statistics underestimate the real population rates, because of the systematic omission of private hospital admission or of admissions to private beds in National Health Service hospitals. Thus, the advantages of using population-based rates are lost if increasing numbers of admissions are ignored. Also, patients who are discharged on the day of admission (day-cases) will often not appear in hospital statistics. Hence, a low rate in a community for hernia repair may mean that a larger proportion are being done as day-cases, not that the use rate is low. Such considerations imply that great care is needed in the interpretation of rates. Similarly, if cross-boundary flow is not accounted for properly, numerators will be inflated by people not at risk of admission in the geographical area.

Inaccuracies in Data Sources

Finally, as well as identified inaccuracies, there may be other kinds which will require careful scrutiny. Thus, completeness of recording all admissions and accurate and reliable population estimates of the appropriate catchment area are obviously essential.

ASSIGNING THE CAUSE TO OBSERVED VARIATION

Thus, any variation observed between populations ought to be a consequence of one or more of these defined reasons. Clearly they each, in principle, interact with one another and it is therefore too simplistic to imagine that they constitute descriptions of discrete mechanisms for variation. However, they do help in understanding what is observed if each is considered as a plausible component taken independently or with others. Broadly speaking, once rates are known to be artefact- and error-free, relate to a coherent catchment (Wennberg and Gittelsohn, 1973) and are age- and sex-standardised, they can be grouped into five categories:

(1) Morbidity.
(2) Random.
(3) Availability and supply.
(4) Clinical.
(5) Demand.

Given the purpose and role of health care, these components have different meanings in terms of their putative role in the causes of variation. Some can be regarded as legitimate, while others are illegitimate or neutral. Morbidity and demand constitute legitimate causes of variation, in the sense that if all variation for a particular cause of admission was determined by variation in morbidity levels and then patient preferences for particular outcomes, then such variation could be wholly appropriate, if commensurate with reasonable public policy and if such preferences did not compromise other, obviously better, choices. On the other hand, if variation is directly caused by variation in supply, method of payment and/or clinical uncertainty, then those responsible for the rational provision of limited health resources will increasingly seek hard justification of the more expensive options. Random variation is inevitable and therefore neutral.

It remains, therefore, to identify the main causes of variation for important reasons for admission to hospital, or for any other medical intervention. Clearly, interventions not routinely recorded will be difficult to test for variation. We shall develop a simple method for distinguishing between these five possible causes.

COMPARING VARIATION

In the USA the (standardised) rate of hysterectomy was around 7–8 per thousand women per year compared with around 1 in Norway, and in the UK it may be nearly 3 (McPherson, 1988). Since such differences clearly have fiscal implications but also health policy implications, such an observation requires investigation. We might, therefore, pursue such an investigation by asking to what extent they can be explained by each of the five broad categories defined above. First, what is known about morbidity differences? In general, this is the first major sticking point in the investigation of causes. For this operation the indications themselves are fairly diverse. Cancer of the uterus and some kinds of invasive cancer of the cervix could give rise to a hysterectomy. Hence, one could compare the incidence of these cancers between the USA, the UK and Scandinavia. Unfortunately this would tell us little about the reasons for the observed differences, because the maximum incidence of these cancers at around age 50–60 is much less than 1 per thousand per year and therefore for all women would be less than 0.1 per thousand per year. The operation is being done much more commonly for other indications (Coulter and McPherson, 1986).

Conditions such as fibroids and menorrhagia are common reasons for the operation. It is, in the present state of routine health statistical information, simply not possible to derive any kind of reliable figure for the incidence of these conditions in these countries. The definition of fibroids or menorrhagia is itself elusive (Chimbira *et al.*, 1980), but even if one knew how to define these things in terms of amount of blood loss or extent of prolapse, it would be difficult to measure the incidence of the conditions for the purposes of comparison. Clearly, it is almost completely logically circular to compare, for instance, consultation rate or admission rates for these conditions, as a proxy for incidence. What is needed are the genuine illness rates uncontaminated by the supply of health resources or the propensity to treat or the desire of the population to seek advice. Hence, population surveys are required and ones which do more than merely ask for a history of symptoms. If a culture has an awareness of heavy periods for some reason, then the number of people reporting these symptoms will be higher than if such things tend to be ignored or suppressed (Coulter *et al.*, 1988).

Thus, in the comparison of hysterectomy rates between countries, an understanding of their cause seems difficult, because the most important potential determinant – morbidity rates – is not measurable. It is not sensible to assume that such differences must be a manifestation of different illness rates, because, as we shall see, there may be no intrinsic difference in morbidity. Moreover, when rates between countries are compared, there are so many other potential reasons for the difference that such comparisons alone are relatively barren from the point of view of understanding their cause. This is because, like morbidity, many of these facets are not easily measurable. Random differences will be small because the numbers of events will be large, but differences in clinical opinion cannot be reliably measured, nor can differences in patient expectation or preferences, because these will necessarily relate to totally hypothetical circumstances. Supply differences often can be reliably measured, but, again, they ought to reflect the supply of facilities and manpower for the procedure being compared, and these will depend on prevailing custom, clinical preferences and patient demand. Hence, comparison between countries, while being of interest and sometimes great fascination, can only be understood when more is known about the reason for the variation, so that some of the many potential causes can be eliminated.

DIFFERENT LEVELS OF POPULATION AGGREGATION

Therefore, it is important to examine the relationship between the above causes and the level of population aggregation to which the rates relate. This is because only through an understanding of this relationship can one begin to discern the dominant causes of variation.

Usually, in terms of routinely available statistics, it is possible to characterise the population at several hierarchical levels. In the British National Health Service, for instance, one can obtain rates nationally, by Regional Health Authority, by District Health Authority and by General Practice. It is also possible to obtain population data by Standard Region or Census District or even by postal code, but these aggregations have a questionable relationship with health provision and therefore a catchment population is more difficult to define and there would be much crossing of these boundaries for health care.

Regions, Districts and GPs, on the other hand, have an obvious relationship with health provision and, hence, the comparison of rates between such aggregations could yield more information. In the first place, taking the smallest aggregation first, we find that over a period of 3 years the (standardised) hysterectomy rate in one practice in Oxfordshire is around 4 per thousand per year but in another it is 1 per thousand per year (McPherson, 1988). In this instance the range of variation seems almost as high as the variation observed between countries, but the explanation might be different. First, since the aggregation level is so much lower, the number of events – even in 3 years – will be low. Therefore, one has to consider chance, or random variation, as a possible explanation. Previously this could not possibly explain the differences between countries, but in this case the rates may only be based on 40 or so operations. This random variation, of course, can be easily tested by conventional significance tests, and if chance is an implausible explanation (i.e. the difference in rates is significant), then we must look for alternative explanations.

In this comparison between small areas the list of potential causes is then much reduced. First, the supply of tertiary hospital services is the same for all GPs, because they all refer their patients to the same hospital with the same consultants. Second, the opportunities for prevailing custom in hospital treatment to differ much between neighbouring GPs is limited. Also, morbidity levels might be expected to be fairly homogeneous, as might patient demand, for, while each practice will differ with respect to social class and other characteristics, since they are all geographically close, such differences are unlikely to be as large as they might be between counties or countries. Hence, the differences in rates are likely to be due to these patient attributes, but most plausibly to differences in the clinical opinion of the GPs themselves, and the way the patient is referred.

It is not immediately obvious that differences in the use rates between neighbouring areas are more likely to be attributable to supply and clinical uncertainty than to characteristics of the patient population, either morbidity levels or perceived utilities of certain outcomes. Yet this distinction is clearly central to the main argument. Its plausibility derives from special studies in which aspects of the populations have been measured (over and above demography) and repeatedly found to have little relationship with use rates, where, on the other hand, supply variables tend to have a strong association (Wennberg and Fowler, 1977). Moreover, a possible determinant of perceived utilities in the UK might be social class, yet very little relationship was observed in a special study of social class and surgical histories (Coulter and McPherson, 1985). This was in spite of social class being often cited as a potent demand factor in the decision-making process. Moreover, Wennberg has argued forcefully that morbidity is unlikely to be a strong determinant of hospitalisation for procedures of high variation between small areas (Wennberg, 1987). An apparent counter-example (McPherson *et al.*, 1985) shows a correlation between cholecystectomy rates and the prevalence of gallstones at autopsy as a measure of morbidity in seven English communities. However, first cholecystectomy exhibits very little variation within the UK (see below) and therefore its indications are agreed upon, but these communities are widely separated all over England, so the homogeneity of neighbouring communities is irrelevant.

SYSTEMATIC, AS OPPOSED TO RANDOM, VARIATION

There is one methodological snag in relation to the further interpretation of utilisation data. Even if the rates between GPs in Oxfordshire are significantly different one from another, there remains an important random component to the variation in rates. Thus, if the international differences in hysterectomy rates range between, say, 7 per thousand and 2 per thousand and similarly the range between GPs is 7–2, such a range does not necessarily imply that the true variations are of similar magnitude. This is important, because the end-product of this inspection of sources of variation is the ability to compare amounts of variation. When we do this, we will want to compare not the variation observed but the real systematic variation there would be if there were no random variation. This is, of course, a contradiction in terms, because to observe anything is to observe with some error. In this context, there is much more error when the number of events is fewer – that is to say, the random error is larger as a proportion of total observed variation and also in absolute terms. The number of events is fewer when the time of observation is short and/or when the population at risk is small and/or when the prevailing rate is low.

Thus, to compare the amount of variation, one has to compare the systematic part of the variation once the random component of variation is removed. To remove the random component, a mathematical form which models the variation process has to be assumed. This is a problem, because such assumptions need not be correct and, hence, the removal of the random component may be biased. As things are, the simplest assumptions are probably the safest and this leads to a simple method for estimating the systematic component of variance. This is described in Appendix 2.1 to this chapter, as well as in McPherson *et al.* (1982).

The model described in Appendix 2.1 assumes that the rates of neighbouring areas vary, not only because of random variation, but also because of systematic differences with regard to all the reasons discussed above. However, this rate is an aggregated statistic and represents the aggregation of all decisions taken in the time period and area of concern. Clearly, therefore, the larger the area the more the rate is aggregated over relevant factors. Thus, a rate for a population of several million will inevitably be the consequence of many doctors and patients making many decisions. On the other hand, the rate for a population of a few thousand will, in general, represent the decisions of many patients but only a few doctors, and therefore may reflect more potently the differences between these few doctors. This is, of course, premised on the assumption that doctors are dominant in the decision-making process – not a controversial view (Wennberg *et al.*, 1982). Hence,

Table 2.1   Plausible sources of variation at different levels of aggregation

Variation between	Morbidity	Supply	Clinical	Demand
GPs	S	O	L	S
Districts	M	M	L	S
Regions	L	L	S	M
Countries	L	L	L	L

L = large; M = medium; S = small; O = no effect relative to others in the same row.

straightforward application of these principles leads to a natural hierar-
chy of plausible causes of observed variation at different levels of
population aggregation. These are shown in Table 2.1. If we use the
above method of measuring variation, then all we are concerned with
will be (1) Morbidity, (3) Supply, (4) Clinical and (5) Demand, because
age and sex are standardised out and the random component will have
been subtracted – if the proportional hazards model is realistic. We now
assume that errors and artefacts are not a problem.

Thus, variations between GPs will be largely a consequence of the
clinical opinions of GPs themselves. Systematic variation between
Districts will be aggregated over GPs but will be a consequence of
variation in consultant opinion and in the supply of facilities, such as
manpower, beds and theatre availability. Variation between regions, on
the other hand, will be the consequence largely of cultural differences in
demand and longstanding differences in the provision of health care,
since the rates will be averaged over many clinical decisions. Almost all
factors could be responsible for variations between countries, which is
one reason why such differences are difficult to interpret, without
ancillary information on causes of variation. This may come from *ad hoc*
studies and from small-area studies.

EXAMPLE FROM COMMON SURGICAL OPERATIONS

If we examine the systematic component of variation for various
procedures at these different levels of aggregation, certain interesting
features appear. In particular, different procedures exhibit totally different patterns of variation, indicating different dominant causes of
variation. The data from which the following calculations are derived are
shown in McPherson (1988). In Table 2.2 the systematic component of
variation is displayed for six surgical operations at different levels of
geographical aggregation (see Appendix 2.2).

Thus, we can see that systematic variation between GPs is often

Table 2.2   Variation between neighbouring areas at different levels of aggregation in England and Wales

Variation between	*Appendicectomy*	*Cholecystectomy*	*Hernia*	*Hysterectomy*	*Prostatectomy*	*Tonsillectomy and adenoidectomy (T and A)*
				Operation		
GPs	6	6	4	6	0	9
Districts	4	4	5	5	6	8
Regions	3	2	4	3	6	5
Countries	7	11	8	11	10	12

higher than it is between districts or regions, suggesting greater differences in the propensity to advise surgery. Prostatectomy is the exception, for which apparently there is no systematic variation between GPs. What this means, of course, is that the variation that is observed is not significantly greater than random variation.

In so far as this variation is a manifestation of clinical differences between GPs, we note that T and A show very high variation; appendicectomy, cholecystectomy and hysterectomy high variation; and hernia repair low variation. This implies that either patient preferences manifested through their choice of GP or GPs' preferences are less consistent for the former operations than for the latter. In particular, they appear to be totally consistent in the recommendation for prostatectomy.

Perhaps more interestingly, the variation between Districts reflects consultant opinion and, therefore, in circumstances of relative homogeneity of provision between neighbouring Districts, largely clinical discretion. If this is the case, then T and As remain the most discretionary, but prostatectomy is now highly variable, presumably reflecting different provision of urologists and disagreements between them in the indications for surgery. It may also be the case that general surgeons perform more or less urological surgery in some Districts. Note that this measure of variation is calculated from data which are independent of those used to calculate the variation between GPs. Of the remaining operations, hernia and hysterectomy are more variable than appendicectomy and cholecystectomy.

We may ask how robust these measures are in relation to changing prevailing rates and to changing circumstances. What do these indices of variation look like in other countries? In Table 2.3 we show the same

Table 2.3 Systematic variation between hospital areas in four countries

	Operation					
Country	*Appendicectomy*	*Cholecystectomy*	*Hernia*	*Hysterectomy*	*Prostatectomy*	*T and A*
England and Wales	4	4	5	5	6	8
Norway	5	4	0	7	7	9
Maine (USA)	4	4	2	6	6	8
Queensland (Australia)	4	–	4	5	6	7

Table 2.4 Age-standardised rates for various procedures by country, per 100 000 per annum

	Operation					
Country	*Appendicectomy*	*Cholecystectomy*	*Hernia*	*Hysterectomy*	*Prostatectomy*	*T and A*
England and Wales	180	80	100	250	90	210
Norway	180	90	200	110	90	110
USA	180	220	280	700	300	310
Australia	280	80	180	450	90	400

statistic for small-area variation in four countries.

To get some idea of the difference in the prevailing rate concealed by these variations within countries, we plot in Table 2.4 the approximate age-standardised rates for each procedure per 100 000 eligible population.

Thus, it can be seen that the actual use of these procedures is, in most cases, quite different between countries, while the small-area variation for each procedure is quite consistent. The main exception to this is hernia repair. This seems to be very much less variable in countries other than England and Wales. At the same time, the operation is much more common in these other countries and there appears to be an inverse relationship between systematic variation and the prevailing rate. This is what might be expected if the higher rates were a manifestation largely of morbidity (which will vary little) and universal access to health care combined with a uniform response to a well-defined set of symptoms. In the case of hernia repair, this explanation is highly plausible, because in the UK some people were still being prescribed non-surgical solutions to their problem. Elsewhere this was not the case and hernia repair was probably available to all who needed it, and inguinal hernias are, of course, easily recognisable.

If one looks at cholecystectomy, on the other hand, several differences emerge. One is that there appear to be low levels of systematic small-area variation in all countries, in spite of large variation between countries. This is probably a manifestation of very different thresholds in circumstances of fiscal constraint compared with fee-for-service systems without effective constraint. In other words, surgical departments functioning within a tight budget will delay gallbladder surgery for any but the most urgent acute cases, while such people in fee-for-service settings may be offered the operation as a prophylaxis against (hypothetical) future problems. In this case the 'correct' indications are clearly totally uncertain, although there is evidence of strong consensus within countries which happen to be set at very different levels, possibly because of supply differences, financial incentives and prevailing custom (McPherson *et al.*, 1985). This is an interesting example of a very-low-variation procedure actually being associated with great uncertainty. Appendicectomy is an example of a low-variation procedure associated with an almost universal consensus – the exception being Australia.

Tonsillectomy was always known to be discretionary from the earliest work of Glover (1938). However, it is not commonly appreciated that prostatectomy and hysterectomy were almost as variable. Hysterectomy is variable at all levels of aggregation, both within and between countries. The fact that the amount of variation decreases as the level of aggregation rises presumably reflects the averaging effect of many decisions. This reflects massive uncertainty about the correct indication for this operation. Indeed there may well be few 'correct' indications and each decision may be an individual matter concerned with finely balanced assessments of anticipated benefits and losses. If this is the case, then such decisions should be made with an eye on the forgone opportunities associated with each marginal hysterectomy. Such operations are then difficult to justify if there is any genuine unmet need elsewhere in the health sector. There is as yet no epidemiological evidence to suggest that hysterectomy rates are to any important extent determined by consumers. There are many medical and other surgical procedures more variable than hysterectomy (Wennberg *et al.*, 1984).

CONCLUSIONS

Such analyses provide insights into the causes of variation of health care decisions which result in the use of hospitals. Most of the 'independent' variables are not themselves very accurately measurable, so assigning causation is particularly problematical. It is not, for instance, possible to measure clinical judgement as a reliable indicator of what clinicians will do. Nonetheless, progress can be made along the lines described. When it is clear that an important component of observed variation is a manifestation of clinical uncertainty, either between GPs, or consultants, or between countries, then assiduous outcome studies ought to be done to measure reliably the utility of different decisions taken on similar patients. The demonstration of uncertainty, in circumstances where certainty is thought to prevail, is only the first step in enlightenment. High rates may be appropriate but, without knowing, it is difficult to justify the expenditure, and, hence, such interventions may be discouraged prematurely. By the same token, the demonstration of a consensus makes the interpretation of utilisation rates much more pertinent for quality assessment. In this case, low rates may well indicate inappropriate neglect of tractable need and high rates a wasteful use of resources.

APPENDIX 2.1

Using the most obvious model to explain differences between regions, a proportional hazard model which is common in epidemiology, leads to the following expression for calculating the systematic component of variation.

If there are k areas between which rates are to be compared, indirect age and sex standardisation, from the overall age- and sex-specific rates, will yield expected numbers of events for each area e_i for the ith area among k. There will be a corresponding observed number of events in the period under study denoted o_i:

$$y_i = \ln\left\{\frac{o_i}{e_i}\right\}$$

Systematic component of variance for y_i:

$$\text{SCV} = \text{var}\left\{\ln\frac{o_i}{e_i}\right\} - \left(\left\{\sum_{i=1}^{k}\frac{1}{e_i}\right\}\middle/k\right)$$

The var (x) means simply the conventional calculation of the variance of

x over all k areas. This assumes that the random error in observed events over and above the systematic variation discussed above is Poisson. Note, however, that the measurement of variance is intrinsically more volatile than measuring means, because single aberrant values of o/e (in this case) will greatly affect the variance of a sample of them. Hence, one should not expect great precision of measurement with anything other than very large samples of areas. Empirical validation by Wennberg (personal communication) seems to suggest that the methodology is sensible and illuminating.

APPENDIX 2.2

In Table 2.2 the systematic component of variation is displayed as:

$$5 \times \ln(100 \times \text{SCV})$$

because the integer value of this number represents a value which is significantly different from neighbouring integers, approximately. Thus, a value of 6 represents a lot of variation, approximately equivalent to the variation seen for hysterectomy between small areas (i.e. approximately a 2–3-fold difference between the highest and lowest rate). Such variation is significantly greater than 5 and less than 7, assuming large sample theory. It should be noted that this index of variation in rates calculated for registerable diseases such as cancer incidence, or for cause-specific mortality, between districts in the UK is rarely greater than unity.

REFERENCES

Aaron, H. J. and Schwartz, W. B. (1984). *The Painful Prescription*. The Brookings Institute, Washington, D.C.

American Child Health Association (1934). The pathway to correction. In *Physical Defects*. New York

Bloor, M. J. and Venters, G. A. (1978). An epidemiological and sociological study of variations in the incidence of operations on the tonsils and adenoids. University of Aberdeen, Institute of Medical Sociology, *Occasional Paper No. 2*

Chimbira, T. H., Anderson, A. B. and Turnbull, A. C. (1980). Relation between measured menstrual blood loss and patient's subjective assessment of loss, duration of bleeding, number of sanitary towels used, uterine weight and endometrial surface area. *Br. J. Obstet. Gynaec.*, **87**, 603–9

Cochrane, A. L. (1972). *Effectiveness and Efficiency: Random Reflections on Health Services*. Nuffield Provincial Hospital Trust, London

Coulter, A. and McPherson, K. (1985). Socioeconomic variations in the use of common surgical operations. *Br. Med. J.*, **291**, 183–7

Coulter, A. and McPherson, K. (1986). The hysterectomy debate. *Q. Jl Social Affairs*, **2**, 379–96

Coulter, A., McPherson, K. and Vessey, M. P. (1988). Do British women undergo too many or too few hysterectomies. *Soc. Sci. Med.*, **27**(9), 897–994

Fitzpatrick, G., Neutra, R. and Gilbert, J. P. (1977). Cost-effectiveness of cholecystectomy for silent gallstones. In Bunker, J. P., Barnes, B. A. and Mosteller, F. (Eds.). *Costs, Risks and Benefits of Surgery.* OUP, Oxford, New York

Gittelsohn, A. and Wennberg, J. E. (1976). On the risk of organ loss. *J. Chron. Dis.*, **29**, 527–35

Glover, J. A. (1938). The incidence of tonsillectomy in school children. *Proc. Roy. Soc. Med.*, **xxxi**, 1219–36

Goldacre, M. and Griffin, K. (1983). *Performance Indicators: A Commentary on the Literature.* Unit of Clinical Epidemiology, University of Oxford, England

Maxwell, R. A. (1981). *Health and Wealth: An International Study of Health Care Spending.* Lexington Books, Lexington, Mass.

OECD (1987). *Financing and Delivering Health Care: A Comparative Analysis of OECD Countries.* OECD, Paris

McPherson, K. (1988). Variations in hospital rates: Why and how to study them. In Ham, C. (Ed.), *Health Care Variations: Assessing the Evidence.* The Kings Fund Institute, London

McPherson, K., Strong, P. M., Jones, L. and Britton, B. J. (1985). Do cholecystectomy rates correlate with geographic variations in the prevalence of gallstones. *J. Epidem. Comm. Hlth*, **39**, 179–82

McPherson, K., Wennberg, J. E., Hovind, O. and Clifford, P. (1982). Small area variations in the use of common surgical procedures: An international comparison of New England, England and Norway. *New Engl. J. Med.*, **307**, 1310–14

Shaw, G. B. (1906). *The Doctor's Dilemma.* In *The Bodley Head Bernard Shaw*, Bodley Head, London, 1971

Wennberg, J. E. (1987). Population illness rates do not explain population hospitalisation rates. *Med. Care*, **25**, 354–9

Wennberg, J. E., Barnes, B. A. and Zubkoff, M. (1982). Professional uncertainty and the problem of supplier-induced demand. *Soc. Sci. Med.*, **16**, 811–24

Wennberg, J. E. and Fowler, F. (1977). A test of consumer contribution to small area variations in health care delivery. *J Maine Med. Ass.*, **68**(8), 275–9

Wennberg, J. E. and Gittelsohn, A. (1973). Small area variations in health care delivery: A population-based health information system can guide planning and regulatory decision making. *Science, N.Y.*, **182**, 1102–9

Wennberg, J. E., McPherson, K. and Caper, P. (1984). Will payment based on diagnosis-related groups control hospital costs? *New Engl. J. Med.*, **311**, 295–300

CHAPTER 3

Variations in Outcomes Research

Leslie L. Roos, Ruth Brazauskas, Marsha M. Cohen and
Sandra M. Sharp

INTRODUCTION

As stressed elsewhere in this volume, the incidence and length of hospitalisation for many surgical procedures and medical conditions vary greatly, both among geographical areas and over time. Although the extent of professional consensus about the need for hospitalisation for a given condition plays a role (Wennberg, 1984; Wennberg *et al.*, 1987a; Roos *et al.*, 1988b), many other factors appear important: bed supply, physician supply and referral patterns. Some of this variation, particularly geographical variation in utilisation with no evidence of variation in population need, may well be medicine which consumes resources but offers no apparent benefit (Roos and Roos, 1981). Other types of utilisation – particularly some of the increased resources going into treatment of the elderly – may be much harder to control (Barer *et al.*, 1987). Because physicians often do not know who is going to die in the short term and who is not, expensive care becomes defensible from both patient and physician perspectives (Scitovsky, 1984, 1985).

Overall, considerable physican activity seems inappropriate according to standards promulgated by panels of expert physicians. Thus, a sizeable percentage of Caesarean sections appears to be inappropriate (Anderson and Lomas, 1984, 1985). Analyses of tonsillectomies and adenoidectomies used data on illness episodes before and after surgery to reach a similar conclusion (Roos *et al.*, 1977; Roos, 1979). RAND researchers have used physician panels to rate the appropriateness of performing different procedures under a number of conditions. Not only did they find a large percentage of procedures performed inappropriately, but also those appropriately performed were only weakly related to an area's overall surgical rate (Chassin *et al.*, 1987; Fink *et al.*, 1987; Winslow *et al.*, 1988a, b).

Patient outcomes form 'one part of the classic triad used to define quality of care: structure, process of care, and outcomes' (Lohr, 1988).

Elements of structure alone, such as a large, well-qualified staff and 'state of the art' equipment, do not guarantee a high level of quality. Outcome evaluations, which measure the impact of care on patients' health status, have received the most attention in recent years. Outcome data by themselves do not indicate how to improve deficiencies in patient care. However, when linked to process information, outcome studies can guide future interventions so that the necessary steps for better care can be implemented (Lohr, 1988).

Concepts of efficacy and effectiveness are critical for outcomes research. Efficacy focuses on the benefit derived by specific individuals having a particular medical problem when medical technology is applied under ideal conditions. Given the discretionary component in most clinical decisions, such technology assessment is essential to reduce physician uncertainty about the advisability of a particular course of action (Caper, 1988). Effectiveness emphasises what a technology actually does. It reflects performance of a medical technology under ordinary conditions when applied by an average practitioner, to a typical patient (Brook and Lohr, 1985). Quality of care may be defined as the difference between efficacy and effectiveness attributed to care providers and their work environment.

The ideal conditions reflected in efficacy versus ordinary conditions defined in effectiveness have their parallels in the methodology of outcomes research. What are the ideal standards for conducting such studies? When circumstances are less than ideal, how can the researcher enhance the reliability and validity of the findings?

Various authors, both in this volume and elsewhere, have stressed the need to develop appropriate methods for the non-experimental study of outcomes (Roper *et al.*, 1988). The first part of this chapter highlights several methodological issues: (1) the various outcome measures; (2) the types of analysis suitable for different kinds of databases; (3) the differences between easily obtained hospital-based data and more desirable population-based data; and (4) advances in risk adjustment.

METHODOLOGICAL ISSUES

Outcome Measures

Some outcome measures require labour-intensive data collection through patient interviews or hospital records review; on the other hand, administrative data, such as insurance claims, provide an excellent source for non-intrusive measures such as readmissions and mortality. Because many databases are maintained and updated for administrative purposes, analyses may be done for a relatively small marginal cost. Outcome measures of quality of care have included the frequently used indicators of mortality and readmission as well as the less familiar 'quality-life years', 'disability-free years' and (particularly for chronic diseases) 'years to remission'. Intervention-free survival has also been used to study surgical outcomes.

Survey measures have been widely used. Their strength lies in providing information on attitudes, feelings and trade-offs; their weakness has been the costs associated with data collection (Fowler et al., 1988). Thus, self-perceived health, ability to perform activities of daily living and ability to live independently in the community are also important for assessing the health status of the general population. Finally, outcome studies focusing on providers generally emphasise patient satisfaction and physician performance standards.

Most of our knowledge pertaining to variation in outcomes is derived from studies using non-intrusive measures. Such measures may be particularly valuable in screening large databases 'to flag events and caregivers with suspect profiles of performance' (Berwick, 1988). Death is easily defined and documented (usually from multiple sources such as death certificates, hospital reports and insurance claims). However, as mortality rates decline, the number of deaths, particularly for single procedures or treatments, becomes very small. Thus, the study of non-fatal events (morbidity) has become more important in recent years, and reflects on quality of life.

Various non-intrusive measures based on claims data are important here:

(1) Short-term readmission to hospital – both within a specified period after surgery and for postsurgical complications. Building upon previous work (Roos et al., 1985), panels of specialists (meeting under the auspices of Health Care Financing Agency in the USA) have developed lists of reasons for readmission which indicate possible complications after a number of common procedures.

(2) Additional surgery after the initial operation.

(3) Long-term problems leading to hospital readmission, such as myocardial infarction and stroke.

(4) Subsequent physician visits with diagnoses indicating continuing problems.

Completeness of the Data

Blumberg (1988) cites the most serious limitation in successfully monitoring outcomes as 'the accuracy, completeness, and relevance of the existing data'. The quality of information from databases must be carefully assessed. Accuracy of the diagnostic data, for example, depends upon both the physicians and the clerks recording the diagnosis. Reflecting the professional training of medical records technicians, diagnoses on hospital records are likely to be more accurate than diagnoses on claims generated by physician visits. Administrative data do not typically include the performance of procedures or laboratory investigations if they are not billable; moreover, the results of such tests are usually not available. Information on risk factors such as smoking and data on drug or other treatments may also not be included.

Some aspects of 'completeness' can determine the design of any study, forming a continuum from relatively simple to relatively complex. Classifying administrative databases by level, at the simplest level (Level 3) only hospital discharge abstracts are needed (Roos and Roos, 1989). Level 3 data can support studies of length of stay and of inpatient mortality; when combined with coverage of a population, such information permits analyses of utilisation across medical market areas. At the intermediate level, Level 2 data require consistent individual identifiers on the hospital discharge abstracts. Hospital claims can be sorted by date and identifying number to generate hospitalisation histories for each individual. Thus, Level 2 data can be used for short-term outcome studies of readmissions and complications after surgery. Such research on quality assurance and cost control can be performed to provide timely feedback to health care institutions. The most comprehensive Level 1 databases possess all the features of the Level 2 and Level 3 files, but include an enrolment file with information for start-up, death and leaving the plan. Longitudinal studies can then follow individuals' health care utilisation through time.

A Level 1 system offering complete coverage for a population can provide both large samples and impressive follow-up capabilities, whether the care be ambulatory, community or hospital-based. The ability to develop individual-based longitudinal histories (both before and after an event or index hospitalisation) permits identifying first-time occurrences in a population. These incident cases represent a more homogeneous group for study; a second operation or recurrence of a condition can be distinguished from new events. As well, the proportion of individuals enjoying 'intervention-free survival' – having no contact with the health care system – can be ascertained.

The Level 1 database of the Health Services Commission in Manitoba, Canada, will be used for many of the examples in this chapter. Medical,

Table 3.1　Data requirements and types of studies using hospital data*

Level	Data requirements	Types of studies
Simple – Level 3	Need hospital discharge abstracts	In-hospital mortality (volume–outcome comparisons, monitoring of individual hospitals); length of stay; small-area analyses
Intermediate – Level 2	Need hospital discharge abstracts and consistent individual identifiers	Timely longitudinal research: short-term readmissions; volume–outcome comparisons, monitoring of individual hospitals; quality assurance and cost control
Comprehensive – Level 1	Need hospital discharge abstracts, consistent individual identifiers, and enrolment file	Highest-quality longitudinal research: short-term and long-term outcome studies; identification of incident cases, volume–outcome comparisons, monitoring of individual hospitals; choice of treatment studies; small-area analysis by person

*From Roos, L. L. and Roos, N. P. Large databases and research on surgery. In Rutkow, I. M. (Ed.), *Socioeconomics of Surgery*. St. Louis, 1989, The C. V. Mosby Co. By permission.

hospital and nursing home care are available to all Manitobans eligible for medical and hospital insurance (with a few exceptions, such as foreign students and armed forces personnel). Because the Commission reimburses out-of-province use and physicians operate under a fee-for-service system, both patients and physicians have an incentive to document utilisation. In addition, the Commission maintains a population-based registry which continually updates the entrance and exit of individuals from the system. Specific checks have established the strong relationship between low use or non-use of the system and good health (Mossey and Roos, 1987).

The Manitoba data also constitute a 'multi-institutional databank' with the capacity to monitor interinstitutional and interphysician variability both in the use of resources and in mortality and rehospitalisation rates (Komaroff, 1985). Longitudinal research, meeting various criteria for high-quality cause-and-effect studies, can be facilitated by such a database (Horwitz, 1987). Thus, the effectiveness of medical practices can be compared on a population-wide basis in a variety of hospitals, not just teaching hospitals. The ability to focus on an individual, a community or the entire population makes this database ideal for assessing health outcomes characterised by major events such as deaths, nursing home admissions and hospitalisations (Roos *et al.*, 1987a). Furthermore, by combining the Manitoba database with other studies, outcomes using the database alone can be compared with outcomes obtained from primary data collection.

Well-organised, high-quality non-experimental databases can support many different types of research, such as analyses of small-area variation, incidence of particular conditions, natural history of illness and efficacy of vaccines. Moreover, research comparing styles, costs and outcomes of care across countries is facilitated by such data. Finally, registries (a necessary part of Level 1 data) may provide information on family relationships – as well as on family formation and dissolution – to aid research in medical genetics.

Population Coverage

Population-based data permit looking at utilisation from an epidemiological perspective, attributing use to individuals according to their place of residence, no matter where the service is provided. Hospital-centred data are generated by individuals visiting one (or more) hospital(s); the population to which these individuals belong is not specified. Despite their convenience, hospital-centred outcome analyses may miss important events in following patients; the outcome variable is typically inpatient mortality. Such research is often limited by the relatively small number of deaths related to specific procedures.

Researchers within the hospital of surgery would seem more likely to pick up readmission or mortality in their own hospital than similar adverse events taking place in other hospitals or outside of hospital. Research covering all utilisation for entire populations has found levels of postsurgical complications and mortality to be considerably higher than those recorded in clinically based studies (Wennberg *et al.*, 1987). Because such findings suggest a lack of complete follow-up in longitudinal studies relying on data from just a single hospital, claims-based cohort research may be the method of choice when large, expensive clinical trials are not feasible.

Risk Adjustment

A major problem in evaluating surgical outcomes across hospitals and physicians has been risk adjustment (Sloan *et al.*, 1986). If patients operated upon at Hospital A have a higher mortality rate and complication rate than patients operated upon at Hospital B, is this because Hospital A's operating team is less skilled? Or is it because the case-mix of patients at the two institutions are different, with Hospital A treating higher-risk patients? One question – with significant implications for studies of quality assurance and cost control – is: when can claims alone be used for these controls and when may prospective data collection be necessary? What sorts of controls would be 'good enough' for testing hypotheses about the relationship between surgical volume and treatment outcomes, for distinguishing the better of two treatments and for identifying hospitals (or physicians) with particularly poor (or especially good) outcomes?

One promising taxonomy for comorbid conditions takes into account not only the number but also the seriousness of comorbid diseases. The comorbidity index of Charlson *et al.* (1987) explained a higher proportion of the variance in 1 year survival rates than a model based solely on the number of comorbid diseases. In a test population with a large set of clinical and demographic variables, age and the comorbidity index were found to be the only two significant predictors of death attributable to comorbid disease.

Computerised hospital admission/separation abstracts can be used to generate covariates, such as the Charlson comorbidity index, for risk adjustment. In the Manitoba research, adding various sorts of other information – claims from physician visits, health status indices from surveys and even some prospectively collected clinical data – provided little additional power in predicting hospitalisation, nursing home entry and mortality (Roos *et al.*, 1988a, 1989).

Manitoba Level 3 data (from the surgical event alone) using age, sex and limited comorbidity information have proved almost as good for risk adjustment as Level 1 data (from both the history of hospitalisations in the preceding 6 months and the surgical event) in predicting mortality and post-surgical readmissions. A model using only prognostic data (comorbidity information from the computerised history preceding surgery), also provided fairly good risk adjustment and similar overall results. Thus, Blumberg's (1986) concerns about using information from the index hospitalisation, rather than prognostic data, do not seem terribly important.

Considerable progress in risk adjustment has been made. If cross-sectional data can accurately identify patients at different degrees of risk, then large-scale studies of inpatient mortality following surgery become relatively easy to conduct; moreover, the published literature comparing outcomes across institutions seems on solid ground (Showstack *et al.*, 1987; U.S. Congress, 1988). The research certainly suggests that useful general covariates can be produced; different covariates need not be generated for each treatment or condition studied (Flood and Scott, 1987; Roos *et al.*, 1989).

THEMES IN THE LITERATURE

Ideally, outcome-based research will assess the health of the entire population of a country, state, county, city or community. This is not always practical; the health status of special subgroups, such as the elderly or low-income groups, is sometimes studied. More typically, outcomes from a single hospital or from an individual clinical department, are assessed. Alternatively, performance at the level of the provider can be reviewed. Finally, the outcomes for specific treatments or alternative treatments can be compared. Outcomes may be short-term or long-term; they may be generated from a single cross-sectional study, from a series of cross-sectional studies or from cohort studies and longitudinal follow-up of specific groups.

The findings and implications of several types of outcomes research are highlighted here. In particular, outcomes may vary: (a) across groups, (b) across treatments, (c) over time, (d) across hospitals and (e) across countries.

Variation in Outcomes Across Groups

The Elderly
One set of studies – the Manitoba Longitudinal Study on Aging – has investigated the elderly's utilisation of medical, hospital, nursing home and home care services, identifying the sociodemographic and health characteristics which increase the risk of specific service use. Interviews from 1975 and 1976 obtained information on sociodemographic, psychosocial, attitudinal and health characteristics of individuals aged 65 and over. Several indices of functional assessment (physical and mental) were part of the interview instrument, and items measuring health status (such as amount of time spent in bed, nearness of relatives and income) were also included. Since the interview data included Manitoba Health Services Commission registration numbers, all health care utilisation (physician visits, hospitalisation, nursing home and home care) was subsequently determined.

Roos and Shapiro (1981) have challenged the assumption that elderly persons use a disproportionately large amount of medical and hospital services. They found that 5% of elderly individuals used 59% of total hospital days utilised by their age group. Most of the elderly enjoyed relatively good health. Reliance on such measures as the number of discharges per thousand population and average length of hospital stay has helped to reinforce the impression that a crisis is looming as the population ages. These Manitoba findings emphasise the importance of identifying the small number of very high users and the reasons for their large consumption of hospital days.

Other research showed that only about 8% of the sample of elderly were admitted to a nursing home in a subsequent 4 year period; of the very elderly (85 years and older), 24% were admitted to a nursing home. An elderly person was more likely to die never having been admitted to a nursing home than he/she was to be admitted (Roos *et al.*, 1984). A third report (Shapiro and Roos, 1984) looked at rural/urban differences in health and health care utilisation. Although no significant differences in health status were found, the rural elderly were more likely to be admitted to hospital and stay there longer than their urban counterparts.

A fourth study looked at non-users of health care – a group of elderly who made no contact with physicians over a 2 year period (Shapiro and Roos, 1985). Non-users tended to be more socially isolated than users; they were more often single, less well educated and more mentally impaired. However, non-users were basically healthy and reported no difficulty in gaining access to physicians. Non-users' mortality and hospitalisation rates for acute care and nursing homes were no different from those who visited physicians. Several reports used the data from the merged files to predict death (Mossey and Shapiro, 1982) and nursing home placement (Shapiro and Tate, 1985).

North American Indians
A recent Manitoba study used readmission algorithms to study complication rates following cholecystectomy for a specific subpopulation – North American Indians (Cohen *et al.*, 1989). Age-specific cholecystectomy rates were highest for young female Natives; whereas the surgical rates have fallen among the rest of the population, rates have remained high for Indian females. The peak age-specific rate was age 30–39 for Indians and age 60–69 for the rest of the population. A multiple logistic regression controlling for age, sex, rural versus urban residence, multiple versus single hospital discharge diagnoses, size of hospital and complex versus simple cholecystectomy was used to assess the risk of readmission to hospital for Natives versus the rest of the population. Natives proved to be 1.46 times more likely to be readmitted to hospital for complications associated with cholecystectomy than were non-Natives. The extent to which this finding holds after application of newer risk-adjusted measures, such as the previously discussed comorbidity index, is a matter of considerable methodological and practical interest.

Variation in Outcomes Across Treatments

Several retrospective cohort studies using Manitoba data have improved our understanding of different treatment alternatives or of long-term complications (Table 3.2). Carrying out such studies using primary data collection would have been quite difficult, owing to loss to follow-up, recall bias and expense. The types of risk-adjustment techniques described earlier have been used to varying extents. In the tonsillectomy analyses, the Manitoba claims data permitted additional controls: unoperated siblings of children having tonsillectomies.

A recent study of tubal ligation provides an example of such research. In order to study whether women having a tubal ligation were at higher risk for menstrual disorders (in some cases necessitating a hysterectomy) (Cohen, 1987), all women who had undergone a tubal ligation in 1974 were selected. A random sample of 10 000 women from the general population of Manitoba in the same age range as the tubal ligation women (25–44) was selected for comparison. All women who had a tubal ligation between 1970 and 1982 or a hysterectomy from 1970 to 1974 were eliminated from the 10 000 sample, leaving two files – women who had, and those who did not have, a tubal ligation in 1974. Women not in the insurance plan over the study period were eliminated from both groups. The two groups of women were compared according to their post-1974 rates of hospitalisation for menstrual disorders, their rates of dilatation and curettage, often used to treat menorrhagia, and their rates of hysterectomy. Short-term adverse gynaecological

Table 3.2 Differences among treatments – claims-based research on outcomes

Problem/treatment	*Results*
Tonsillectomy:	
Operate versus not operate	Similar to those in clinical trial; clarified when procedure likely to be helpful, noted frequency of inappropriate use (Roos *et al.*, 1977; Roos, 1979)
Infective endocarditis:	
Medical versus surgical treatment	Close to a 'toss-up' between treatments; suggested usefulness of clinical trial, limited picture of longer-term outcomes provided (Abrams *et al.*, 1988)
Prostatectomy:	
Open versus transurethral (TURP)	Results indicated open procedures may have benefits over transurethral procedures; good picture of long-term outcomes provided (Roos and Ramsey, 1987; Wennberg *et al.*, 1987; Roos *et al.*, 1989)

outcomes were similar between women who had undergone a tubal ligation and the comparison women. However, over an 8 year period, women aged 25–29 at the time of their tubal sterilisation had 1.6 times the risk of hysterectomy after controlling for previous gynaecological history, marital status and number of physician visits and hospitalisations. For women over 30, tubal sterilisation was not a risk factor for subsequent hysterectomy in either the short or the long term.

Variation in Outcomes over Time

Technological change and changes in technique may be responsible for some improvements in outcomes over time. Given the initial mortality rates, considerable improvements in the results of coronary artery bypass graft surgery have been reported. Both Yeaton and Wortman (1985), in a meta-analysis, and Pryor *et al.* (1987), using the Duke Data Base for Cardiovascular Disease, found improved results over time with bypass surgery. The Duke researchers, who have risk-adjusted for baseline prognostic factors, report relatively little postsurgical morbidity (Pryor *et al.*, 1987; Bounous *et al.*, 1988).

A study of adverse outcomes of surgery in Manitoba for the period 1972–83 highlights some additional issues. The growth over this decade in centralisation of high-risk procedures and in the proportion of procedures performed by high-volume specialists was associated with slightly reduced adverse outcomes for hysterectomy, cholecystectomy and prostatectomy. Changes were revealed in both the types of patients coming to surgery and the types of procedures performed, so that declines in rates of readmission may relate to more general changes in the health care system rather than to an actual decrease in postsurgical complications. Moreover, such external factors as resource availability can influence medical decision making. For example, postsurgical admission rates may decline as a result of a decrease in availability of beds – not necessarily a change in quality of care (Roos *et al.*, 1987b).

Variation in Outcomes Across Hospitals and Practitioners

A number of studies have shown that, even after controlling for as many variables as feasible, wide interhospital differences in the rates of poor outcomes can be expected (Luft *et al.*, 1979; Wennberg *et al.*, 1987b). The most-researched and most-supported proposition explaining these results is the 'volume–outcome' hypothesis: surgical outcomes are better in hospitals with relatively high volumes of the given procedure.

Can such scholarly research have an impact? Risk-adjusted outcome data presented by Steinbrook (1988) showed wide hospital-by-hospital variation in California inpatient mortality rates after coronary artery bypass surgery (and several other procedures). Relevant *Los Angeles Times* articles identified the rates at individual hospitals. Steinbrook (1988) notes that the bypass findings, in particular, 'triggered wide discussion within the medical community throughout the state'. Such data should also make it possible for patients (consumers of health care) to consider their hospital of surgery very carefully.

Such procedure-specific data may have more of an impact than the overall mortality rate data published by Health Care Financing Agency (HCFA) in the USA. Vladeck *et al.* (1988) report that publication of the HCFA 'death list' did not appear to 'discourage consumers (be they patients or physicians who admit patients) from continuing to use hospitals with poor outcomes'. Both looking for variation at the individual surgeon level (rather than the hospital level) and examining charts of survivors and decedents in high- and low-mortality-rate hospitals would appear useful. Identifying specific and measurable components of quality and developing a system to evaluate and monitor them have been proposed (Caper, 1988). The California data certainly highlight the need for such work.

Variation in Outcomes across Countries

Comparisons across countries add several dimensions to outcome studies. Given the wide range in outcomes among hospitals, international differences might depend primarily on the distribution of good and poor hospitals in various countries. Alternatively, structural differences in the delivery of care among nations might be responsible for observed differences. Replication of results comparing treatments in more than one country supports the generalisability of any differences; because details of treatment may vary somewhat across countries, results duplicated internationally are more convincing than results confirmed within a single country (Roos *et al.*, 1989).

Cross-national comparisons provide an important perspective on the cost–quality relationship. On the one hand, medicine's image as a science-based discipline may have 'created expectations among the public, as well as within the medical profession, that standards for quality in medicine could be more rigorously defined than may be the case in other disciplines' (Caper, 1988). On the other hand, Shortell and Hughes (1988) have warned that American hospitals 'facing both greater regulatory or payment constraints and a highly competitive market may be most likely to have poorer patient outcomes'. The relationship of cost control to quality of care is illuminated by comparative data. If, for example, Canadian data were to show that the same, or better, outcomes could be obtained at considerably less cost than in the USA, the feasibility of saving funds by adopting some of the strategies of another country could be examined. The dialogue of cost control and quality assurance might change noticeably.

Outcome Differences: Suggested Research

Combining extensive population-based data with in-depth data from one or more settings may prove particularly useful in exploring why poor outcomes may result. Which factors are most important?

In recent Manitoba work, all anaesthetic encounters at a large tertiary-care teaching hospital from 1975 to 1983 were included in a database containing information on preoperative medical conditions, preoperative drug usage and a preoperative assessment of the patient's clinical condition using the American Society of Anesthesiologists' (ASA) physical status score (1 = healthy normal, 5 = not expected to live beyond 24 h, even with surgery) (Saklud, 1941). The ASA physical status score was an excellent predictor of intraoperative and postoperative complications associated with anaesthesia and surgery (Cohen and Duncan, 1988). Information on demographics (such as age and sex) and mortality as well as specific procedures and discharge diagnoses was provided through linkage to the Manitoba Health Services Commission and the provincial Vital Statistics databases (Cohen et al., 1986).

Patients having a pre-operative medical condition were found to be at much higher risk of having a postoperative complication (within 48 h of the procedure); the risk for a postoperative complication was highest in the organ system with the preoperative problem (Duncan and Cohen, 1987). Surgical mortality rates did not decrease over time after controlling for age, sex, physical status and type of surgical procedure. Furthermore, the contribution of anaesthesia to mortality was not significant as compared with patient and surgical factors (Cohen et al., 1988).

The linkage of the anaesthesia follow-up data with claims data also facilitates several new types of outcome studies.

First, data on experience of an anaesthesiologist can be incorporated into the more standard analyses considering the surgeon's experience and hospital volume as independent variables affecting the outcomes of common surgical procedures (U.S. Congress, 1988). Will the negligible effect of anaesthesia variables on outcomes described above hold, controlling for specific type of surgery? This type of study should provide valuable information on one element of 'process'.

Second, inpatient morbidity after each common surgical procedure can be examined and related to postsurgical morbidity leading to complication and readmission to hospital. Such research is important both for its own sake and for assessing the importance of concerns that using diagnoses on claims from a hospitalisation for surgery will seriously confuse presurgical and postsurgical morbidity (Blumberg, 1986). Large-scale studies of inpatient morbidity are relatively rare, owing to the costs involved (Charlson and Sax, 1987; Charlson *et al.*, 1987; Flood and Scott, 1987). We are aware of no studies relating inpatient postsurgical morbidity to postsurgical readmissions after the initial hospitalisation.

Alternative Interpretations

Might something other than quality of care account for observed, risk-adjusted variation in outcomes among providers, areas, and so forth? Our knowledge as to what is responsible for these outcome differences is incomplete.

Perhaps differences in patient selection unaccounted for by the risk-adjustment process are responsible. The ability to specify covariates or predict outcomes may vary considerably across specialties; cardiology may be the best-developed specialty in this regard. Thus, researchers using the Duke Data Base for Cardiovascular Disease (Pryor *et al.*, 1985; Hlatky *et al.*, 1988) have forwarded a number of risk factors available in claims databases:

(1) History of myocardial infarction, cardiomegaly, congestive heart failure.
(2) History of, or concurrent, angina.
(3) Type of angina.
(4) History of disease affecting heart valves.
(5) History of, or concurrent, cerebral or peripheral vascular disease.
(6) Age.
(7) Sex.

Other more clinically detailed prognostic risk factors (such as a measure of the left ejection fraction) are lacking in claims data. The extent to which such clinically detailed variables provide predictive information beyond that more readily available from claims needs to be assessed. Ongoing work at Health Care Financing Administration in the USA is addressing this problem. Flood and Scott (1987) found that several somewhat more general measures did not contribute additional predictive power.

Other variables have been suggested. Patient ethnicity or socioeconomic status may be an independent predictor beyond measured illness-related variables (Berkman and Breslow, 1983; Marmot, 1986). Physiological measures (such as the APACHE score) may provide additional predictive power (especially for very ill patients). Considerable work could be done here; however, substantial evidence suggests that these additional factors *cannot* account for the magnitude of the differences observed in effectiveness studies (Flood and Scott, 1987).

Randomised clinical trials are an alternative, often a 'gold standard' alternative, to cohort or case controls in studying efficacy. Such trials do help resolve questions of risk adjustment. However, clinical trials have not been used for research on effectiveness; individuals have not been randomly assigned to hospitals or physicians. Such trials seem unlikely.

The importance of diagnostic data suggests the need for better understanding of differences in recording or diagnosing. Because hospital abstracters may differ in style, the impact of interhospital differences in the number of diagnoses recorded might be minimised by using just each patient's primary diagnosis for research purposes (Blumberg, 1986). However, indices (such as the Charlson comorbidity index) often risk-adjust by incorporating secondary diagnoses from the hospitalisation for surgery. Thus, considerable information is lost by not using these data. The bias imparted or statistical power gained by using all the diagnoses on the hospital discharge abstract can be examined empirically. Checks on recording can be made by independent chart review. Differences in diagnostic choice among physicians are harder to deal with. Various studies have shown a fair degree of disagreement among physicians (Koran, 1975; Dubois *et al.*, 1987); resolving such differences in chart review may be time-consuming or impossible.

Efficacy versus Effectiveness

Although clinicians need to be able 'to measure and compare the benefits and risks of various preventive, diagnostic, therapeutic, or rehabilitative approaches' (Laupacis *et al.*, 1988), well-designed efficacy studies characteristically show few differences among treatments. Improvements due to innovative therapies in surgery and anaesthesia are usually relatively modest: '. . . 4 out of 10 innovations in secondary therapy produce a reduction in complication rates of 10% or more, while 2 or 3 out of 10 innovations in primary therapy produce a 5% or greater increase in survival' (Gilbert *et al.*, 1977).

On the other hand, cohort studies often find a fourfold or greater range in risk-adjusted postsurgical mortality among hospitals (Wennberg *et al.*, 1987b; Steinbrook, 1988). Clearly, much more attention should be paid to variations in outcomes among hospitals and physicians. Patients may not benefit as much when surgery is performed at hospitals with relatively poor outcomes. From this perspective, effectiveness may be more important than efficacy; clinicians, patients and policy makers know how these benefits and risks vary in the real world of physicians and hospitals.

DISCUSSION

What should be done to improve outcomes research? How can it be changed to be more relevant to policy makers? The impact of actual or potential changes in utilisation on quality (and patient outcomes) could be partially monitored in a system that would incorporate adjusted mortality indicators, statistical analysis of these indicators and selection of a sample of deaths (not necessarily just outliers) for process-of-care review. Brook and Lohr (1987) suggest that this would permit evaluators to identify outliers and to examine trends by time period and by geographical area, across all diagnoses and for individual diagnoses.

The lack of data showing benefits flowing from high levels of service has led to pressures for changes in delivery. Hospitals delivering services to regions with very high levels of utilisation are natural targets for planners with budgetary responsibilities. Are there some general tactics for studying the effects of changes in delivery? Level 3 data will facilitate before–after studies showing any shifts in where residents of a given catchment area receive their treatment: is there a change in general and specific utilisation from one hospital to another? How great is any change from hospital-based to ambulatory treatment? Have bed closures had any effect? Regions or catchment areas where no new programmes or structural changes have taken place can serve as control groups.

The longitudinal perspective implicit in individual-based (Level 1) data can facilitate comparisons of:

(1) The outcomes of specific types of ambulatory versus in-patient surgery, controlling for case-mix.

(2) The outcomes of treatment for particular medical conditions, controlling for case-mix. Although the reliability and validity of medical diagnoses need considerable work, major interhospital differences in outcomes of medical admissions have been shown (Dubois *et al.*, 1987). Preliminary work with the Manitoba database has shown similar interhospital variation, variation greater than is characteristically found for surgical outcomes.

Monitoring changes in specific practices (and outcomes) targeted by the budget in conjunction with examining changes in overall utilisation (to provide controls) would permit estimating the effects of various structural changes.

Other issues might be studied in analogous fashion. For example, the effects of such changes as those in physician supply might be studied, using such measures as:

(1) The percentage of the elderly and other high-risk groups receiving vaccination for influenza.

(2) The percentage of each age group having pap smears and the history of pap smears in the period before diagnosis of cervical cancer.

(3) The percentage of each age group having mammography and the history of mammography in the period before diagnosis of breast cancer.

(4) The percentage of individuals with stroke having no diagnosis of hypertension in the previous 6 months.

(5) The management of diabetes according to accepted standards.

The tracers suggested above differ in the extent to which the efficacy of the suggested treatment has been established; different activities may or may not be appropriate for various age groups. Thus, among the elderly, the efficacy of vaccination to prevent influenza may be greater than that of pap smears and mammography for elderly detection of cancer (Strassburg *et al.*, 1986; Battista and Grover, 1988). Effectiveness data from a population base have been generally lacking. Although research on each of the above tracers would have to be tailored to the particular issues surrounding the preventive or treatment strategy, the potential is clear. Outcomes studies can be extended beyond their current emphasis on morbidity and mortality.

Organisations of institutions and providers need to become more involved in an educational process. In addition to sharing techniques and software associated with screening and checking, a senior manager in each state or province should have responsibility for training technicians and auditing results. Blumberg (1988) has advocated giving an independent high-level group the 'responsibility of certifying that an outcome model is sufficiently useful to be applied under specified circumstances'.

Lohr *et al.* (1988) have stressed the importance of standardisation: '. . . medical record keeping is local and uses practice-specific terminology; this fragmentation means that information on diagnosis, treatment, and outcomes cannot be linked across settings.' Standardisation would permit those responsible (public or private insurers, the Colleges of Physicians and Surgeons in Canada) to carry out the data analysis; then the appropriate agencies can follow up on poor outcomes. For example,

Blumberg (1988), in discussing how to make effective use of data already routinely included in computerised hospital abstracts, suggests the further development of coding manuals to ensure uniformity.

Co-operation between those collecting primary data and those using claims would also help. If researchers doing in-depth clinical studies would specifically include some measures present in claims data, checks on risk adjustment and outcomes would be greatly facilitated. Population-based data must be centralised at a state, provincial or national level to permit analyses which capture both the original hospital admission and readmission to the hospital of surgery or to a hospital different from the first. At the same time, data must be accessible. The monitoring and feedback process presupposes co-operation among health care institutions, clinicians and researchers.

Hospitals typically are not in as good a position as insurers in terms of having access to all the data used to prepare outcome statistics. Blumberg (1988) suggests that 'hospitals will have to be able to request and obtain more specific reports from the organisation to follow up on hunches they may have regarding the cause of disparities between observed and expected outcomes'.

Such efforts are under-way. In Manitoba the Health Services Commission supports a Management Information Section to make specific runs for hospitals and other relevant agencies interested in undertaking analyses. Many of the runs relate to variations across areas and length of stay by drug-related groups (DRGs), but an output format suitable for use by hospitals has been designed. Hospitals need only to specify: procedures and diagnoses of interest, whether they wish to receive inpatient mortality data or data at a specified interval after surgery. In addition to overall statistical results to be produced on demand for each hospital, individual cases with information as to diagnosis, attending physician, surgery, and so forth, can be produced. This can facilitate hospital-based quality assurance committees' efforts to look at their own cases in greater detail. Appropriate hospital records can then be pulled, enabling the committees to focus on particular problems. Management Information Section staff have been kept busy making runs; such activity seems likely to increase.

In summary, deficiencies in the delivery of health care have been well documented. An epidemiology of quality has been advocated: 'just as we will continue to explore and document variations in per capita use of services across the nation, we will need to know how quality is distributed in the population' (Brook and Lohr, 1985). In the USA the Health Care Financing Administration (HCFA) has undertaken a major initiative to assess medical technology, using data from the Medicare systems of claims processing and peer review to 'monitor trends and assess the effectiveness of specific interventions' (Roper *et al.*, 1988).

Such work oriented towards improving outcomes is encouraging; one component of the initiative emphasises feedback to practitioners. Perhaps actual improvement in outcomes will follow.

ACKNOWLEDGEMENTS

The authors gratefully acknowledge the help of the Manitoba Health Services Commission. The preparation of this chapter was supported by National Health Research and Development (Canada) Project No. 6607–1197–44. Interpretations and viewpoints contained in this chapter are the authors' own and do not necessarily represent the opinion of either the Manitoba Health Services Commission or Health and Welfare Canada. The authors also wish to thank Kerry Meagher for the preparation of the manuscript. Some of this material has appeared in I. M. Rutkow (Ed.), *Socioeconomics of Surgery*, C. V. Mosby Co., St. Louis, M., 1988.

REFERENCES

Abrams, H. B., Detsky, A. S., Roos, L. L. and Wajda, A. (1988). Is there a role for surgery in the acute management of infective endocarditis? A decision analysis and medical database approach. *Medical Decision Making*, 8, 165–74

Anderson, G. M. and Lomas, J. (1984). Determinants of the increasing cesarean birth rates – Ontario data 1979 to 1982. *New England Journal of Medicine*, 311, 887–92

Anderson, G. M. and Lomas, J. (1985). Explaining variations in cesarean section rates: patients, facilities or policies? *Canadian Medical Association Journal*, 132, 253–9

Barer, M. L., Evans, R. G., Hertzman, C. and Lomas, J. L. (1987). Aging and health care utilization: new evidence on old fallacies. *Social Science and Medicine*, 24, 851–62

Battista, R. N. and Grover, S. A. (1988). Early detection of cancer: an overview. *Annual Review of Public Health*, 9, 21–45

Berkman, L. F. and Breslow, L. (1983). *Health and Ways of Living: The Alameda County Study*. Oxford University Press, New York

Berwick, D. M. (1988). Toward an applied technology for quality measurement in health care. *Medical Decision Making*, 8, 253–8

Blumberg, M. S. (1986). Risk adjusting health care outcomes: a methodologic review. *Medical Care Review*, 43, 351–93

Blumberg, M. S. (1988). Measuring surgical quality in Maryland: a model. *Health Affairs*, 7(1), 62–78

Bounous, B. P., Mark, D. B., Pollock, B. G., Hlatky, M. A., Harrell, F. E., Lee, K. L.

Rankin, J. S., Wechsler, A. S., Pryor, D. B and Califf, R. M. (1988). Surgical survival benefits for coronary disease patients with left ventricular dysfunction. *Circulation* (Suppl. I), **78**, 151–7

Brook, R. H. and Lohr, K. N. (1980). *Quality Assurance in Medical Care: Lessons from the U.S. Experience.* The Rand Corporation, Santa Monica, Calif.

Brook, R. H. and Lohr, K. N. (1985). Efficacy, effectiveness, variations, and quality: boundary-crossing research. *Medical Care*, **23**, 710–22

Brook, R. H. and Lohr, K. N. (1987). Monitoring quality of care in the Medicare program: two proposed systems. *Journal of the American Medical Association*, **258**, 3138–41

Caper, P. (1988). Defining quality of medical care. *Health Affairs*, **7**(1), 49–61

Charlson, M. E., Pompei, P., Ales, K. L., MacKenzie, C. R. (1987). A new method of classifying prognostic comorbidity in longitudinal studies: development and validation. *Journal of Chronic Diseases*, **40**, 373–83

Charlson, M. E. and Sax, F. L. (1987). The therapeutic efficacy of critical care units from two perspectives: a traditional cohort approach vs. a new case-control methodology. *Journal of Chronic Diseases*, **40**, 31–9

Chassin, M. R., Kosecoff, J., Park, R. E., Winslow, C. M., Kahn, K. L., Merrick, N. J., Keesey, J., Fink, A., Solomon, D. H. and Brook, R. H. (1987). Does inappropriate use explain geographic variations in the use of health care services. *Journal of the American Medical Association*, **258**, 2533–7

Cohen, M. M. (1987). Long-term risk of hysterectomy after tubal sterilization. *American Journal of Epidemiology*, **125**, 410–19

Cohen, M. M. and Duncan, P. G. (1988). Physical status score and trends in anaesthetic complications. *Journal of Clinical Epidemiology*, **41**, 83–90

Cohen, M. M., Duncan, P. G., Pope, W. D. B. and Wolkenstein, C. (1986). A survey of 112,000 anesthetics at one teaching hospital (1975–83). *Canadian Anaesthesiology Society journal*, **33**, 22–31

Cohen, M. M., Duncan, P. G. and Tate, R. B. (1988). Does anesthesia contribute to operative mortality? *Journal of the American Medical Association*, **260**, 2859–63

Cohen, M. M., Young, T. K. and Hammarstrand, K. H. (1989). Ethnic variation in cholecystectomy rates and outcomes, Manitoba, 1972 to 1984. *American Journal of Public Health*, **79**, 751–755

Dubois, R. W., Rogers, W. H., Moxley, J. H. and Brook, R. H. (1987). Hospital, inpatient mortality: Is it a predictor of quality? *New England Journal of Medicine*, **317**, 1674–80

Duncan, P. G. and Cohen, M. M. (1987). Postoperative complications: factors of significance to anaesthetic practice. *Canadian Journal of Anaesthesiology*, **34**, 2–8

Fink, A., Brook, R. H., Kosecoff, J., Chassin, M. R. and Solomon, D. H. (1987). Sufficiency of clinical literature on the appropriate uses of six medical and surgical procedures. *Western Journal of Medicine*, **147**, 609–14

Flood, A. B. and Scott, W. R. (1987). *Hospital Structure and Performance.* Johns Hopkins University Press, Baltimore

Fowler, F. J., Wennberg, J. E., Timothy, R. P., Barry, M. J., Mulley, A. G. and Hanley, E. (1988). Symptom status and the quality of life following prostatectomy. *Journal of the American Medical Association*, **259**, 3018–22

Gilbert, J. P., McPeek, B. and Mosteller, F. (1977). Progress in surgery and anesthesia: benefits and risks of innovative therapy. In Bunker, J. P., Barnes,

B. A. and Mosteller, F. (Eds.), *Costs, Risks, and Benefits of Surgery*. Oxford University Press, New York, pp. 124–69

Hlatky, M. A., Califf, R. M., Harrell, F. E., Lee, K. L., Mark, D. B. and Pryor, D. B. (1988). Comparison of predictions based on observational data with the results of randomized controlled clinical trials of coronary artery bypass surgery. *Journal of the American College of Cardiologists*, **11**, 237–45

Horwitz, R. I. (1987). The experimental paradigm and observational studies of cause-effect relationships in clinical medicine. *Journal of Chronic Diseases*, **40**, 91–9

Komaroff, A. L. (1985). Quality assurance in 1984. *Medical Care*, **23**, 723–34

Koran, L. (1975). The reliability of clinical methods, data, and judgments. *New England Journal of Medicine*, **293**, 642–6, 695–701

Laupacis, A., Sackett, D. L. and Roberts, R. S. (1988). An assessment of clinically useful measures of the consequences of treatment. *New England Journal of Medicine*, **318**, 1728–33

Lohr, K. N. (1988). Outcome measurement: concepts and questions. *Inquiry*, **25**, 37–50

Lohr, K. N., Yordy, K. D. and Thier, S. O. (1988). Current issues in quality of care. *Health Affairs*, **7**(1), 5–18

Luft, H. S., Bunker, J. P. and Enthoven, A. C. (1979). Should operations be regionalized? The empirical relation between surgical volume and mortality. *New England Journal of Medicine*, **301**, 1364–9

Marmot, M. G. (1986). Epidemiology and the art of the soluble. *Lancet*, **1**, April 19th, 897–900

Mossey, J. M. and Roos, L. L. (1987). Using claims to measure health status: the illness scale. *Journal of Chronic Diseases* (Suppl. 1), **40**, 41S–50S

Mossey, J. M. and Shapiro, E. (1982). Self-rated health: a predictor of mortality among the elderly. *American Journal of Public Health*, **72**, 800–8

Pryor, D. B., Califf, R. M., Harrell, F. E., Hlatky, M. A., Lee, K. L., Mark, D. B. and Rosati, R. A. (1985). Clinical databases – accomplished and unrealized potential. *Medical Care*, **23**, 623–47

Pryor, D. B., Harrell, F. E., Rankin, J. S., Lee, K. L., Muhlbaier, L. H., Oldham, H. N., Hlatky, M. A., Mark, D. B., Reves, J. G. and Califf, R. M. (1987). The changing survival benefits of coronary revascularization over time. *Circulation* (Suppl. V), **76**, V13–V21

Roos, L. L. (1979). Alternative designs to study outcomes: the tonsillectomy case. *Medical Care*, **17**, 1069–87

Roos, L. L., Cageorge, S. M., Austen, E. and Lohr, K. N. (1985). Using computers to identify complications after surgery. *American Journal of Public Health*, **75**, 1288–95

Roos, L. L., Nicol, J. P. and Cageorge, S. M. (1987a). Using administrative data for longitudinal research: comparisons with primary data collection. *Journal of Chronic Diseases*, **40**, 41–9

Roos, L. L. and Roos, N. P. (1989). Using large data bases for research on surgery. In Rutkow, I. M. (Ed.), *Socioeconomics of Surgery*. Mosby, St. Louis, Mo., pp. 259–75

Roos, L. L., Roos, N. P. and Sharp, S. M. (1987b). Monitoring adverse outcomes of surgery using administrative data. *Health Care Financing Review* (Suppl.), **7**, 5–16

Roos, L. L., Sharp, S. M. and Cohen, M. M. (1989). Risk adjustment in claims-based research: the search for efficient approaches. *Journal of Clinical Epidemiology*, to be published

Roos, N. P., Henteleff, P. D. and Roos, L. L. (1977). A new audit procedure applied to an old question: Is the frequency of T & A justified? *Medical Care*, **15**, 1–18

Roos, N. P. and Ramsey, E. (1987). A population-based study of prostatectomy: long term outcomes associated with differing surgical approaches. *Journal of Urology*, **137**, 1184–8

Roos, N. P. and Roos, L. L. (1981). High and low surgical rates: risk factors for area residents. *American Journal of Public Health*, **71**, 591–600

Roos, N. P., Roos, L. L., Mossey, J. M. and Havens, B. J. (1988a). Using administrative data to predict important health outcomes: entry to hospital, nursing home, and death. *Medical Care*, **26**, 221–39

Roos, N. P. and Shapiro, E. (1981). The Manitoba Longitudinal Study on Aging: preliminary findings on health care utilization by the elderly. *Medical Care*, **19**, 644–57

Roos, N. P., Shapiro, E. and Roos, L. L. (1984). Aging and the demand for health services; Which aged and whose demand? *Gerontologist*, **24**, 31–6

Roos, N. P., Wennberg, J. E. and McPherson, K. (1988b). Using diagnosis-related groups of studying variations in hospital admissions. *Health Care Financing Review*, **9**, 53–62

Roos, N. P., Wennberg, J. E., Malenka, D., McPherson, K., Anderson, T., Cohen, M. M. and Ramsey, E. (1989). Mortality and reoperation following open and transurethral resection of the prostate for benign prostatic hypertrophy. *New England Journal of Medicine*, **320**, 1120–24

Roper, W. L., Winkenwerder, W., Hackbarth, G. M. and Krakauer, H. (1988). Effectiveness in health care: An initiative to evaluate and improve medical practice. *New England Journal of Medicine*, **319**, 1197–1202

Saklud, M. (1941). Grading of patients for surgical procedures. *Anesthesiology*, **2**, 281–5

Scitovsky, A. A. (1984). The high cost of dying: what do the data show? *Milbank Memorial Fund Quarterly*, **62**, 591–608

Scitovsky, A. A. (1985). Changes in the costs of treatment of selected illnesses, 1971–1981. *Medical Care*, **23**, 1345–57

Shapiro, E. and Roos, L. L. (1984). Using health care: rural/urban differences among the Manitoba elderly. *Gerontologist*, **24**, 270–4

Shapiro, E. and Roos, N. P. (1985). Elderly non-users of health care services; their characteristics and their health outcomes. *Medical Care*, **23**, 247–57

Shapiro, E. and Tate, R. B. (1985). Predictors of long-term care facility use among the elderly. *Canadian Journal on Aging*, **4**, 11–19

Shortell, S. M. and Hughes, E. F. X. (1988). The effects of regulation, competition, and ownership on mortality rates among hospital inpatients. *New England Journal of Medicine*, **318**, 1100–7

Showstack, J. A., Rosenfeld, K. E., Garnick, D. W., Luft, H. S., Schaffarzick, R. W. and Fowles, J. (1987). Association of volume with outcome of coronary artery bypass graft surgery: scheduled vs. nonscheduled operations. *Journal of the American Medical Association*, **257**, 785–9

Sloan, F. A., Perrin, J. M. and Valvona, J. (1986). In-hospital mortality of surgical patients: Is there an empiric basis for standard setting? *Surgery*, **99**, 446–53

Steinbrook, R. (1988). Hospital quality in California. *Health Affairs*, **7**(3), 235–6

Strassburg, M. A., Greenland, S., Sorvillo, F. J., Lieb, L. E. and Habel, L. A. (1986). Influenza in the elderly: report of an outbreak and a review of vaccine effectiveness reports. *Vaccine*, **4**, 38–43

U.S. Congress, Office of Technology (1988). *The Quality of Medical Care: Information for Consumers*. OTA-H-386, Government Printing Office, Washington, D.C.

Vladeck, B. C., Goodwin, E. J., Myers, L. P. and Sinisi, M. (1988). Consumers and hospitals: the HCFA 'Death List'. *Health Affairs*, **7**(1), 122–5

Wennberg, J. E. (1984). Dealing with medical practice variation: a proposal for action. *Health Affairs*, **3**(2), 6–32

Wennberg, J. E., Roos, N. P., Sola, L., Schori, A. and Jaffe, R. (1987). Use of claims data systems to evaluate health care outcomes: mortality and reoperation following prostatectomy. *Journal of the American Medical Association*, **257**, 933–6

Winslow, C. M., Kosecoff, J. B., Chassin, M., Kanouse, D. E. and Brook, R. H. (1988a). The appropriateness of performing coronary artery bypass surgery. *Journal of the American Medical Association*, **260**, 505–9

Winslow, C. M., Solomon, D. H., Chassin, M. R., Kosecoff, J., Merrick, N. J. and Brook, R. H. (1988b). The appropriateness of carotid endarterectomy. *New England Journal of Medicine*, **318**, 722–7

Yeaton, W. H. and Wortman, P. M. (1985). The evaluation of coronary artery bypass graft surgery using data synthesis techniques. *International Journal of Technology Assessment in Health Care*, **1**, 125–40

CHAPTER 4

Medical Decision Making and Practice Variation

Albert G. Mulley, Jr.

INTRODUCTION

Wide variations in the application of medical technologies have recently become the object of intense scrutiny and debate. Much of the attention has been motivated by the evident implications of such variations for the quality and cost of medical care (Wennberg and Gittelsohn, 1982). But these variations also raise serious questions about the process of clinical decision making for patients, physicians, those with responsibility to gather and disseminate information on which clinical decisions are based, and health policy makers. The focus on the decision-making process has been sharpened by the professional uncertainty hypothesis (Wennberg *et al.*, 1982). This hypothesis holds that when geographical variation cannot be explained by differences in disease prevalence, access to and availability of services, or enabling factors such as insurance, it reflects differences in physicians' beliefs about the value of the variable procedures and practices for meeting patients' needs. The uncertainty may result from inadequate information on the part of some professionals when the information is known to others, or may reflect the real limits of medical knowledge at the time (Eddy and Billings, 1988). The stochastic nature of biological systems guarantees that, even with full information, medical decisions will always include an element of risk.

Practice variation, *measured from case to case*, may reflect differences in valuations made by different people (or *for* different people) for the same health outcomes. When the purpose of the intervention is to improve the quality of life, preferences and underlying values may be the critical variables in determining whether the procedure is indicated or not. Such variability is desirable and should be preserved. For most variable procedures and interventions, it is unlikely that the populations' distributions of preferences for relevant outcomes are sufficiently different to explain observed variation. More likely, providers in areas with different rates have different preferences and/or attitudes towards risk, and their views (overly) influence the decision; the agency role is inadequate for the complex communication tasks necessary to allow adequate definition of patient preferences so that the choice made will be consistent with the relevant utilities and attitudes towards risk (Wennberg *et al.*, 1988; Mulley, 1989).

Decision analysis (also termed prescriptive decision theory, to distinguish it from descriptive decision theory, which is described below) is a systematic approach to decision making under conditions of uncertainty (Raiffa, 1968; Weinstein and Feinberg, 1980). The method requires careful consideration of the structure of a decision problem, including the logical and temporal sequence of acts and contingent events. The method also requires explicit, quantitative treatment of uncertainty (using Bayesian or subjective probabilities) and explicit quantitative treatment of values (using utility theory). The central premise is that the rational decision maker would (if he or she could) adhere to axioms of the expected utility model. The structured and quantitative nature of decision analysis avoids the traps that result from counterintuitive relationships between independent and conditional probabilities. The explicitness of decision analysis forces the revelation of, and distinction between, what is known and not known (and the degree of confidence) and what is valued and not valued.

Decision analysis can, therefore, be invaluable in understanding controversies and in distinguishing between practice variations that reflect uncertainty, whether avoidable or not, and those that reflect differences in values. It can help in establishing relative priorities for information gathering (e.g. to better define effectiveness) and for information dissemination to improve the function of the professional agency role.

Descriptive decision theory defines the *is* rather than the *ought to be* of decision making, including medical decision making. Empirical evidence points to predictable deviations from the rational model (Kahneman *et al.*, 1982; Kassirer *et al.*, 1987; Pauker and Kassirer, 1987). What can be predicted can often be avoided or, at least, understood well enough to avoid the consequences of poor decisions.

The purpose of this chapter is not to provide a primer of decision analysis or descriptive decision theory or a review of methodological issues. Such primers and reviews are available (Weinstein and Feinberg, 1980; Kahneman *et al.*, 1982; Hershey and Baron, 1987; Kassirer *et al.*, 1987; Pauker and Kassirer, 1987). Rather, the objective is to consider how prescriptive and descriptive decision theory can be used by those who would understand and respond constructively to practice variation. I shall argue that the more explicit approach to decision making embodied by decision analysis not only forces a distinction between questions of information and questions of values, but also clarifies the decision-making responsibilities of physicians, patients and those health policy makers who set the context in which clinical decisions are made. The argument can be exemplified in the clinical field as follows.

PRESCRIPTIVE DECISION THEORY: THE PROSTATECTOMY DECISION

The following clinical scenario may help us to understand the role of decision analysis in understanding practice variation.

> A 72-year-old man, married and sexually active, has had increasing symptoms of bladder irritation and urethral obstruction due to benign prostatic hypertrophy (BPH). He gets up twice each night to void and during the day he voids frequently with a sensation of urgency. He relates these symptoms to a primary care physician, who refers him to a urologist, who in turn recommends a transurethral prostatectomy (TURP). Should he have the procedure? If so, who should pay for it?

It is evident that the decision must be made in the face of considerable uncertainty and ambiguity. Symptoms of BPH have diminished the man's quality of life. Surgery is likely to relieve symptoms and thereby improve quality but the result could be no important improvement or even a worsening of symptoms. Furthermore, surgery involves the risk of a complication resulting in incontinence, impotence or even death.

The uncertainty and ambiguity can be reduced by referring to collective past experience: what have been the rates of symptom improvement, surgical complications and operative mortality among similar patients who chose TURP, and what was the course of symptoms for those who didn't? Presumably, the patient would want the best possible estimates of the likelihood of symptom deterioration or improvement, incontinence, impotence or death, with or without TURP. But it is evident that the right choice for the individual will depend as much or more on values as on probabilities. Men with the same level of prostatic symptoms, measured objectively, might experience very different degrees of functional limitations, discomfort and worry about health due to the condition of their prostate. Therefore, the decision hinges not only on a complex sequence of probabilistic events, but also on trade-offs between quantity and quality of life and between different attributes of health which variably define quality for different people.

If our patient or his doctor were a decision analyst, he or she might approach this complex task by defining objectives in terms of valued health outcomes, including length of survival and determinants of

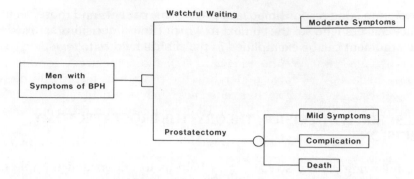

Figure 4.1 A simple decision tree representing a choice (indicated by the square node) between watchful waiting, for which the short-term outcome is continued moderate symptoms of BPH, and prostatectomy, which confers a chance (indicated by the round node) of either improvement to mild symptoms, a surgical complication or death

quality of life, and available choices. A logical structure of events contingent on each choice would be developed to link any choice to the outcomes of concern. In its simplest form, the decision structure could be represented by a decision tree which depicts the choice between surgery, i.e. a gamble between improvement and a complication resulting in worsening or death, and no surgery or 'watchful waiting', which, in this simplified version, means that the patient will have to live with his symptoms (Figure 4.1). More elaborate trees could be constructed which would include the possibility of different complications of surgery as well as allow for spontaneous improvement or worsening of symptoms which may convince the patient to 'cross over' from watchful waiting to surgery. What is known about the therapeutic and adverse effects of TURP would be expressed explicitly and quantitatively in the form of probabilities. The relative value of possible outcomes, ideally reflecting the well-considered judgements of the patient who would live (or die) with the outcome, would be expressed explicitly and quantitatively in the form of utilities. The product of such an analysis would be the expected utility, or expected benefit, for each available alternative. The expected utility of TURP, less the expected utility of the alternative with the highest expected utility (e.g. 'watchful waiting'), would be the *net expected utility* of TURP. If the net expected utility were positive, the decision analyst's patient would presumably undergo TURP; if the net expected utility were negative, he would not.

Such an analysis of the prostatectomy decision has been performed; it provides a sense of both the potential and the limitations of decision analysis (Barry *et al.*, 1988). The analysis was based on an elaborate model including Markov processes to approximate the course following

TURP and watchful waiting. Probability estimates were derived from: (a) a critical review of the literature (Barry, 1987); (b) analysis of claims data to provide less biased estimates of objective outcomes such as operative mortality (Wennberg *et al.*, 1987); and (c) a survey conducted among patients who have undergone the procedure to provide more accurate estimates of subjective outcomes, such as functional status and symptom level (Fowler *et al.*, 1988). Utility estimates for these outcomes were derived from the expert opinions of urologists. Any estimates other than those of a particular patient who must make a choice and live with the consequences should be recognised as arbitrary.

The analysis produced a number of insights into the two clinical theories that underlie most decisions to perform TURP: (a) that the surgery extends life expectancy by reducing the likelihood of complications of prostatism and doing so at a time when the patient is younger than if it were deferred and therefore less likely to suffer operative complications; and (b) that surgery relieves stable but bothersome symptoms of prostatism and thereby improves the quality of life. These insights stem from a better understanding of the elements of the net expected benefit of TURP.

Without adjustments of the outcomes for quality considerations based on symptoms and functional status, the net expected benefit of TURP is negative. That is, operative mortality associated with prostatectomy more than outweighs the combined risks of death due to complications of chronic urinary retention associated with BPH, increased mortality associated with emergent rather than elective procedures, and the increased operative mortality associated with the comorbidity of older age when the surgery is deferred. The results of the analysis indicate, therefore, that for most men with prostatism, TURP should not be performed to improve survival.

The patient survey data indicate that there are a large number of relevant functional states that affect quality and must be considered if outcomes are to be fully described. These include increasing degrees of obstructive and irritative symptoms as well as incontinence and sexual dysfunction (Fowler *et al.*, 1988). Even more important, the survey demonstrates the need to consider individual patients' preferences for well-specified outcomes. While impotence may be considered terrible by some men, a significant number of those who report not having erections when stimulated do not consider the erectile dysfunction a 'problem'. Clearly, the former group risk more than the latter when submitting to elective prostatectomy.

When utilities are used to quality-adjust future years faced by men with stable symptoms of prostatism, the operative strategy has a positive net expected benefit for many. Surgery is favoured by a positive trade-off between life expectancy (greater with watching) and the

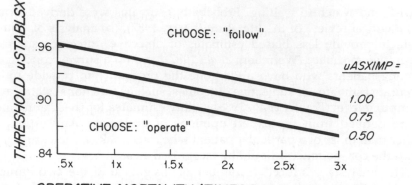

Figure 4.2 The threshold utility of moderate symptomatic prostatism (ustablsx) as it varies with operative mortality and with the utility associated with impotence. Patients in the lower left corner, with low operative mortality and poor quality of life because of their symptoms, should choose surgery. Those in the upper right corner, with high operative mortality and less decrease in quality of life due to symptoms, should choose watchful waiting. The more life's quality is diminished by impotence (the lower the uasximp) the more constrained the indications for surgery. From Barry *et al.* (1988)

expected quality of life. Multiple-sensitivity analyses indicate that operative mortality and the degree of disutility associated with the stable symptom state are the most important variables in assessing net expected benefit for the individual patient. The three-way sensitivity analysis, reproduced as Figure 4.2, can be used to identify indications and contraindications for surgery, using estimates of these two variables. The diagonal lines of Figure 4.2 indicate those circumstances for which net expected benefit is zero. Each line represents a different degree of disutility associated with impotence. If operative mortality is lower and/or the utility of life with symptoms is less (i.e. the symptoms are perceived as worse), the net expected benefit is positive. If mortality and utility are greater than the pairs represented by the diagonals, the net expected benefit of surgery is negative and the procedure is contraindicated.

Returning to our hypothetical patient, we can consider how he might use the results of such an analysis. Assuming that the base case probabilities used in the analysis apply to him, and that he is interested in length of life rather than quality (as far as it is diminished by symptoms of prostatism), he should forgo surgery to avoid a loss of life expectancy. If, however, he is willing to lose some life expectancy to rid himself of symptoms, and the utilities used in the analysis are also applicable, he will have a net gain in quality-adjusted life expectancy with TURP. He might wonder whether he can lower his operative risk by treating some comorbid conditions before surgery, or seeking out a 'better' hospital or surgeon. He might consider just how much he is bothered by his current symptoms and quantify that utility relative to those of other possible outcomes, such as impotence. By doing so and referring to Figure 4.2, he could judge whether either surgery or watchful waiting represents a good bet (whether his utility and operative mortality place him close to the origin or in the right upper corner of Figure 4.2) or more of a toss-up, where the choice is more ambiguous and might be influenced by the utility of impotence or by attitudes towards risk and other variables not fully accounted for in the analysis.

HOW REALISTIC IS THE DECISION-ANALYTIC APPROACH?

There is a neatness and precision about the construction of models, the calculation of net expected benefit and the display of sensitivity analyses, that reflect both the strengths and weaknesses of decision analysis. It has been shown repeatedly that clinicians communicate about uncertainty, among themselves and with patients, with a great deal of imprecision. Qualitative terms like 'possibly', 'rarely', 'almost certainly' etc. are used to avoid getting committed to the precision of a probability estimate. These terms are however, context-specific and interpreted very differently by different people (Bryant and Norman, 1979; Kong *et al.*, 1986). Even when precise probability estimates are rendered, there are problems in using these probabilities to make the 'right' clinical choices (Berwick *et al.*, 1981; Eddy and Billings, 1988). The task of probability revision, using new diagnostic information, or other tasks that require an understanding of conditional probabilities, can be hazardous for clinicians at all levels of training (Casscells *et al.*, 1979).

The explicit estimation of utilities as well as probabilities forces a clear distinction between questions of information and questions of values. For the thoughtful analyst, it also raises important questions about the different roles and responsibilities for clinical decision making and provides a reminder that patient utilities should be paramount. But precise value judgements are even more difficult to render than precise probability estimates. Utility assessment methods have evolved from both the economic and psychometric traditions and have been used extensively to measure utility for health states (Mulley, 1989). But serious questions remain about measurement validity or even the approach to defining validity. Scepticism about utility assessment has been fuelled by evidence that utilities for some health states vary widely not only among individuals (Sackett and Torrance, 1979; McNeil *et al.*,

1981), as might be expected, but also with the format used for describing the health state (Llewellyn-Thomas *et al.*, 1982), the framing of the outcomes (Tversky and Kahneman, 1981), the outcomes used to anchor the scale (Sutherland *et al.*, 1983), the scaling task used (Read *et al.*, 1984) and other situation-specific factors (Ciampi *et al.*, 1982). A clinician, or anyone who must make value-laden decisions on a regular basis, would not be surprised. He or she may view a utility as a precisely rendered opinion – an important opinion if it serves as the basis for a clinical decision or resource allocation, but an opinion nonetheless. Opinions may be mindful or mindless. They may reflect deeply held values, but they also reflect what we know and what we can imagine. Opinions may differ depending on who is asking, how they are asking, and how we think our answers will be perceived and used. And opinions change. The stark contrast between the quantification and precision of utilities and the qualitative and often ephemeral nature of value judgements represents the biggest challenge in applying formal decision analysis to medical decision making.

Even if we could be confident in our ability to estimate probabilities and assess utilities, we would still be obliged to question the underlying assumptions of the approach. Decision analysis relies fundamentally on the expected utility model, which in turn is based on axioms of rational choice (Von Neumann and Morgenstern, 1947; Raiffa, 1968; Hershey and Baron, 1987). People do not behave in accordance with these axioms. For example, patients may be averse to making choices that involve risk of a bad outcome and prefer an outcome with a utility less than the expected value of the risky alternative. Descriptive decision theory describes the *is* of decision making and distinguishes it from the *ought* prescribed by prescriptive theory. Common heuristics used when making choices have been defined which often lead to 'irrational' or 'illogical' decisions (Kahneman *et al.*, 1982). Well-documented non-linearities in utility functions which differ for gains and losses make the choice of reference points and framing of outcomes critically important determinants of decision-making behaviour. Such non-linearities of utilities, combined with equally prevalent non-linearities in the way people actually weigh outcomes with probabilities, i.e. overweighing small probabilities and underweighing mid-range probabilities, form the basis for prospect theory (Kahneman and Tversky, 1982). But it is important to recognise that descriptive decision theory is not concerned with the description of decision-making behaviour for its own sake. Rather, descriptive theory is directed at defining deviations from the normative model that is the basis for decision analysis so that corrections can be made of either decision makers or the normative model (Hershey and Baron, 1987).

DECISION ANALYSIS AND THE RIGHT RATE QUESTION

While the calculation of the expected net benefit of TURP may help an individual to decide whether or not to undergo surgery, how does it help a policy maker to respond to the observed wide variation in prostatectomy rates across geographic areas that are otherwise apparently similar? How can the expected net benefit help to determine the answer to the question: which rate is right? The question can be considered in an abstract sense by focusing on the familiar cost–benefit curve in Figure 4.3. For this example, the number of times a particular procedure such as TURP is performed in a population of a fixed size (e.g. 100 000) is measured along the horizontal axis and the *aggregate* benefit derived from the procedure is measured along the vertical axis. It is assumed that individual patients vary, because of different clinical circumstances and personal preferences, in how much they can benefit from the procedure and that those with greater expected benefit receive the procedure before those with less expected benefit. As Figure 4.3 is drawn, marginal benefits decrease with additional use, eventually reaching a rate (point F) at which additional procedures produce no benefit and begin to do more harm than good, detracting from the aggregate benefit.

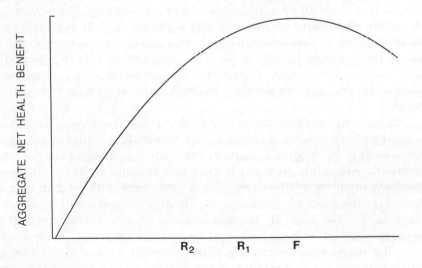

Procedures/100,000

Figure 4.3 Aggregate net health benefit as a function of number of procedures performed in a population of fixed size. Marginal benefits decrease with additional use, reaching zero at point F (full care). Lower levels of use that imply rationing of the procedure and health benefits are indicated by points R_1 and R_2

A policy maker with access to the information represented in Figure 4.3 could make some well-informed judgements about preferred procedure rates. For the policy maker concerned only about the aggregate benefit derived from TURP, there is a right rate, represented by point F. The policy maker who also cared about costs, or the total benefits derived from not only TURP, but also other procedures and health care activities to which resources might be diverted from TURP, would certainly want to avoid any rates higher than F but might prefer a lower rate, such as R_1 or R_2, to cut cost or to divert resources to alternative uses with higher marginal benefits, with a view to increasing the efficiency of care.

How does this abstraction relate to the individual clinical decision and the concept of net expected benefit? Figure 4.4 brings us a bit closer to the clinical perspective. The number of procedures is again represented on the horizontal axis, but the vertical axis indicates benefits *per procedure*. This figure makes more explicit the variable benefit assumptions that underlie the more familiar shape of Figure 4.3: high benefits may accrue when the procedure is strongly indicated and performed with low risk, but other patients in other circumstances may expect a low level of benefit, or even harm. It is important to recognise that the downward-sloping line in Figure 4.4, which underlies the decreasing slope in Figure 4.3, suggests not only that some patients benefit less than others from the same procedure, but also that there is an effective triage mechanism. Without effective triage, the procedure might be performed in patients with low or negative net expected benefit (i.e. expected harm) before it is performed in those with a high net expected benefit. The curve in Figure 4.3 would undulate and, perhaps, even repeatedly cross the horizontal axis, if patients were treated as they presented, somewhat randomly, rather than by rank order according to expected benefit.

Clinical decisions could easily be made, within the constraints established by policy makers, if the necessary information were available and formulated as in Figure 4.4. Some number equal to or less than F would receive the procedure, how much less being determined by the stringency of any rationing of these procedures made necessary by their cost or desirable diversion of resources to alternative uses. But Figure 4.4 remains, for the clinical decision maker, an unrealistic abstraction because of the difficulty in defining the vertical axis. The difficulty stems from the necessity of estimating clinical benefit *a priori* in the face of multiple uncertainties and difficult value judgements. As we have seen, the decision analysts' solution to the problem is to calculate the net expected benefit. It is this measure of benefit which captures the uncertainty as well as information, and values as well as outcomes and which, therefore, most appropriately defines the vertical axes of Figures 4.3 and 4.4.

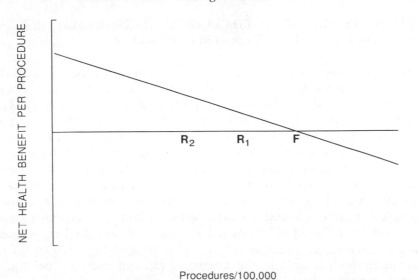

Procedures/100,000

Figure 4.4 The net health benefit per procedure. Points F, R_1 and R_2 correspond to the same points on Figure 4.3

It is apparent that different kinds of variables determine what the net expected benefit of TURP, or any other intervention, may be for an individual patient. The skill of the surgeon and/or others involved in performing the procedure may vary, increasing or decreasing the probability of complications or death. The patient's risk of a bad outcome, with or without the procedure, may be influenced by illness unrelated to BPH or other target conditions. The probability of improved outcome, with or without the procedure, may be influenced by discernible clinical characteristics; diagnostic assessment may be useful to focus on appropriate probabilities of outcomes for a particular patient. These considerations would sound familiar to the clinician who would weigh risks and benefits using the same formulation implicitly. But, as already noted, even when probabilities for the same outcomes – defined precisely by means of physical, psychological and social function – are identical for patients, their expected benefit may be different because of different preferences or utilities. These utilities may be strongly influenced by the patient's baseline status and needs as well as attitudes and beliefs. Differences in any of these variables that determine net expected benefit – either probabilities or utilities – should lead to variation in use of procedures and medical practices which is entirely appropriate. Decision analysis can help both clinicians and policy makers to distinguish that variation which should be preserved because it represents personal or cultural preferences from that which represents avoidable ignorance, uncertainty or failure of the rational agency model.

PROSPECTS FOR IMPROVED CLINICAL DECISION MAKING: RECOGNISING THE LOCI OF RESPONSIBILITY

The need for better information about outcomes of medical interventions has become the focus of attention for researchers and policy makers concerned about the implications of practice variation (Wennberg *et al.*, 1980, 1982, 1988; Wennberg and Gittelsohn, 1982; Eddy and Billings, 1988; Ellwood, 1988; Roper *et al.*, 1988). However, as noted in the introductory chapter of this volume, outcome information is a necessary but not sufficient element of any strategy designed to respond constructively to problems in medical practice which may contribute to observed variations. From the decision theorists' perspective, a more complete strategy would include steps to improve access to and organisation of available knowledge and measures to help clinical decision makers to avoid errors in reasoning and logic which reflect unwitting deviations from the axioms of rational decision making. A complete strategy would also include steps to ensure a decision process that paid due respect both to the importance of individual patients' preferences and to societal interests that justify, depending on circumstances, both the promotion and the constraint of clinicians' and patients' decision-making autonomy. Any such strategy must recognise the complexity of medical decision making. Any implementation plan must recognise that the complexity is increased by the necessary sharing of the responsibility for clinical decision making among clinicians, patients and policy makers who act as societal agents.

Clinicians as Professional Agents

Clinicians have the responsibility to maintain an accurate and organised information base and use that information to inform patients and help them make informed decisions. It is a prodigious task, which becomes more difficult with each advance in medicine's scientific base and could become ever more difficult with the needed explosion of information on outcomes. Clinical information must be compiled in a manner that facilitates its discriminating use. Problems with the internal and external validity of clinical studies must be recognised. Methods for discriminating electronic retrieval of the medical literature must be improved (Haynes *et al.*, 1986; Ad Hoc Working Group for Critical Appraisal, 1987). The large clinical databases proposed as a response to variations (Wennberg *et al.*, 1980; Ellwood, 1988; Roper *et al.*, 1988) should be constructed in a manner that facilitates clinically relevant subgroup analyses and thereby facilitates accurate estimation of probabilities.

Information to estimate probabilities better will be wasted if clinicians cannot improve their ability to revise probabilities and otherwise reason probabilistically. Repeated demonstrations of mistaken logic cannot be dismissed as academic esoterica. While limited rationality (Simon, 1979) of decision making can be documented in many disciplines, few make decisions that so profoundly affect the quantity and quality of life as do physicians. More self-conscious examination of the hypothetico-deductive method and other approaches to clinical decision making must become a focus for educational reform in medical schools and in clinical practice.

Clinicians do far more than provide and process information. They use their collected vicarious experience to help patients to value possible outcomes of medical care. Here the difficult task is to predict how patients would feel when they reach a health state they can only imagine (Mulley, 1989). They also help patients to understand the context of any risks associated with medical interventions. Communication of subjective experiences and risks, and elicitation of the respective preferences and attitudes, are inherently difficult. But, again, seldom is it so profoundly important as in the decision shared by doctor and patient. Clinical scientists must build new theories that focus on the shared nature of clinical decision making which sometimes escapes the descriptive decision theorists' single-actor perspective. The irreducible difference in perspective between rational agent and client must be recognised if we are to understand the implications of deviations from the normative model of decision making. For example, deviations from the normative model based on a minimax regret strategy (avoiding a choice that has a higher expected utility because it includes a possibility of the worst outcome) may be appropriate if it is the patient's concern about regret that drives the decision, but may not be if it reflects the physician's concern about responsibility and associated regret for a bad outcome that follows an intervention rather than one that 'just happens'. The role of negotiation and bargaining between doctors and patients has been widely examined (Balaint, 1957; Stoeckle, 1987). It is a role that is changing with the changing expectations of the participants (Stoeckle, 1989). This work needs to be more explicitly integrated with the work of normative and descriptive decision theorists.

Patients as Clients

Patients must recognise the complexity of the role that they play in the process just described. Foremost, they must accept the responsibility that comes with any desired level of decision-making autonomy. They should appreciate that protection from such responsibility, and the associated anxiety and potential regret, can be provided by the physician who takes a more paternalistic approach (Thaler, 1980; Hershey and Baron, 1987). But if the paternalistic decision is to reflect the patient's values and attitudes towards risk, those values and attitudes must be communicated. Too much variation in values and attitudes, among patients and between doctors and patients, has been documented to assume concordance.

While patients must accept responsibility either for decision making or for the communication of preferences, exercise of that responsibility generally must follow some education about options and outcomes from the provider. Often the process is iterative and time-consuming. New educational technologies, including interactive video disc programming, have the potential to provide more efficiently the educational context for informed, shared decision making (Wennberg et al., 1988).

Societal Agents

Policy makers who represent societal interests have the responsibility to provide the organisational context in which good decision making can proceed. Decision makers are often shielded from immediate financial considerations by public or private insurance mechanisms. Public health education provides a basis for some health care decisions. National libraries and databases exist, and, in many countries, policy makers are responding to mandates, based on concerns about costs and quality, to improve availability of information (Roper et al., 1988).

Any long-term strategy by policy makers to deal with practice variation should focus on ways to improve physician–patient decision making. Policy makers should resist the temptation to use consensus-based criteria for care as a quick fix to potential cost or quality problems associated with variations (Mulley and Eagle, 1988). Such criteria may be useful in the short term to target extreme practices for review and as a measurement standard. However, there is a real risk that such criteria could codify practices that reflect current consensus but that have not been adequately tested. More important, the consensus process requires consensus judgements about values as well as probabilities. Even carefully assembled consensus groups may not adequately represent appropriate societal values. Demonstrated variability in patient prefer-ences for at least some outcomes should temper promulgation of doctrinaire approaches to clinical problems.

Policy makers also have the responsibility to set constraints for health care decisions. Some decisions may be constrained by a society's widely shared ethical precepts. More decisions are constrained by resources. Whether nations or communities are spending 5% or 15% of their resources on health care, they could extend their budget limitations and still spend more on programmes with a positive expected benefit. Forgoing such expenditures constitutes rationing. The manner in which such rationing is accomplished has major implications for practice variation and for the efficiency and equity of health services. These issues are addressed in the following two chapters.

REFERENCES

Ad Hoc Working Group for Critical Appraisal (1987). A proposal for more informative abstracts of clinical articles. *Ann. Int. Med.*, **106**, 598–604

Balaint, M. (1957). *The Doctor, the Patient and the Illness*. International University Press, New York

Barry, M. J. (1987). Determining the effectiveness of surgery for benign prostatic hypertrophy. In, Wennberg, J. E., *Assessing Outcomes for Patients with Hypertrophy of the Prostate*. Report to the National Center for Health Services Research and Health Care Technology Assessment. Department of Health and Human Services/Public Health Service

Barry, M. J., Mulley, A. G., Fowler, F. J. *et al.* (1988). Watchful waiting vs. immediate transurethral resection for symptomatic prostatism: The importance of patients' preferences. *J. Am. Med. Ass.*, **259**, 3010–17

Berwick, D. M., Fineberg, H. V. and Weinstein, M. C. (1981). When doctors meet numbers. *Am. J. Med.*, **71**, 991–8

Bryant, G. D. and Norman, G. R. (1979). Expressions of probability: Words and numbers. *New Engl. J. Med.*, **302**, 411

Casscells, W., Schoenberger, A. and Graboys, T. B. (1978). Interpretation by physicians of clinical laboratory results. *New Engl. J. Med.*, **299**, 999

Ciampi, A., Silberfeld, M. and Till, J. E. (1982). Measurement of individual preferences: the importance of situation-specific variables. *Med. Decision Making*, **2**, 483

Eddy, D. M. and Billings, J. (1988). The quality of medical evidence: implications for quality of health care. *Hlth Aff.*, **7**(1), 19–32

Ellwood, P. M. (1988). Outcomes management: a technology of patient experience. *New Engl. J. Med.*, **318**, 1549–56

Fowler, F. J., Wennberg, J. E., Timothy, R. P. *et al.* (1988). Symptom status and quality of life following prostatectomy. *J. Am. Med. Ass.*, **259**, 3018–22

Haynes, R. B., McKibbon, A., Fitzgerald, D. *et al.* (1986). How to keep up with the medical literature. V. Access by personal computer. *Ann. Int. Med.*, **105**, 810–24

Hershey, J. L. and Baron, J. (1987). Clinical reasoning and cognitive processes. *Med. Decision Making* **7**, 203

Kahneman, D., Slovic, P. and Tversky, A. (Eds.) (1982). *Judgement under Uncertainty: Heuristics and Biases*. Cambridge University Press, Cambridge

Kahneman, D. and Tversky, A. (1982). The psychology of preferences. *Sci. Am.*, **246**, 160

Kassirer, J. P., Moskowitz, A. J., Lau, J. and Pauker, S. G. (1987). Decision analysis: A progress report. *Ann. Int. Med.*, **106**, 275–91

Kong, A., Barnett, G. O., Mosteller, F. and Youtz, C. (1986). How medical professionals evaluate expressions of probability. *New Engl. J. Med.*, **315**, 740–4

Llewellyn-Thomas, H., Sutherland, H. J., Tibshirani, R., Ciampi, A., Till, J. E. and Boyd, N. F. (1988). The measurement of patients' values in medicine. *Med. Decision Making*, **2**, 449

McNeil, B. J., Weichselbaum, R. and Pauker, S. G. (1981). Speech and survival: Tradeoffs between quantity and quality of life in laryngeal cancer. *New Engl. J. Med.*, **305**, 982

Mulley, A. G. Jr. (1989). Assessing patients' utilities: Can the ends justify the Means? *Med. Care*, **27**, S269–S281

Mulley, A. G. Jr. and Eagle, K. A. (1988). What is inappropriate care? *J. Am. Med. Ass.*, **260**, 540–1

Pauker, S. G. and Kassirer, J. P. (1987). Decision analysis. *New Engl. J. Med.*, **316**, 250–8

Raiffa, H. (1968). *Decision Analysis: Introductory Lectures on Choice under Uncertainty*. Addison-Wesley, Reading, Mass.

Read, J. L., Quinn, R. J., Berwick, D. M. *et al.* (1984). Preferences for health outcomes: comparisons of assessment methods. *Med. Decision Making*, **4**, 315

Roper, W. L., Winkenwerder, W., Hackbarth, G. M. and Krakauer, H. (1988). Effectiveness in health care: An initiative to evaluate and improve medical practice. *New Engl. J. Med.*, **319**, 1197–202

Sackett, D. L. and Torrance, G. W. (1978). The utility of different health states as perceived by the general public. *J. Chron. Dis.*, **7**, 347

Simon, H. A. (1979). Information process models of cognition. *Ann. Rev. Psych.*, **30**, 363–96

Stoeckle, J. D. (1987). Tasks of primary care. In Goroll, A. H., May, L. A. and Mulley, A. G. Jr. (Eds.), *Primary Care Medicine*, 2nd edn. Lippincott, Philadelphia

Stoeckle, J. D. (1989). Reflections on modern doctoring. *Milbank Mem. Fund Q.* (in press)

Sutherland, H. J., Dunn, V. and Boyd, N. F. (1983). Measurement of values for states of health with linear analogue scales. *Med. Decision Making*, **3**, 477

Thaler, R. (1980). Toward a positive theory of consumer choice. *J. Econ. Behav. Organiz.*, **1**, 39

Tversky, A. and Kahneman, D. (1981). The framing of decisions and the psychology of choice. *Science, N.Y.*, **211**, 453

Von Neumann, J. and Morgenstern, O. (1947). *Theory of Games and Economic Behavior*. Princeton University Press. Princeton, N.J.

Weinstein, M. C. and Feinberg, H. V. (1980). *Clinical Decision Analysis*. Saunders, Philadelphia

Wennberg, J. E., Barnes, B. A. and Zubkoff, M. (1982). Professional uncertainty and the problem of supplier-induced demand. *Soc. Sci. Med.*, **16**, 811–24

Wennberg, J. E., Bunker, J. P. and Barnes, B. (1980). The need for assessing the outcome of common medical practices. *Ann. Rev. Publ. Hlth*, **1**, 277–95

Wennberg, J. E. and Gittelsohn, A. (1982). Variations in medical care among small areas. *Sci. Am.*, **246**, 120–34

Wennberg, J. E., Mulley, A. G. Jr., Hanley, D. *et al.* (1988). An assessment of prostatectomy for benign urinary tract obstruction: Geographic variations and

the evaluation of medical care outcomes. *J. Am. Med. Ass.*, **259**, 3027–30
Wennberg, J. E., Roos, N., Sola, L. *et al.* (1987). Use of claims data systems to evaluate health care outcomes: Mortality and reoperation following prostatectomy. *J. Am. Med. Ass.*, **257**, 933–6

CHAPTER 5

Equity and Variability in Modern Health Care

Gwyn Bevan

INTRODUCTION

This chapter explores the relationships between medical practice variation and geographical equity in health care. To do so it is necessary to define what is meant by each term. As this chapter shows, despite the importance of equity to most societies, there is considerable confusion about what this means and lack of clarity over which objective is actually sought in accepting equity as an objective of government policy. Therefore, one of the first tasks of this chapter is to define equity and its relationship to different kinds of medical practice variation.

The existence of medical practice variation may be due to various causes, many of which are not directly the result of discretion by physicians. Physicians can only treat those who present themselves for treatment (although they can have some influence over this) with the resources at the physician's disposal. Accepting these constraints on physicians, there clearly is scope for variation in treatment: i.e. different physicians may treat similar patients (with similar conditions and the same entitlement to treatment) differently. Even the same physician may treat similar patients differently because the patients' preferences are different. Are such differences inequitable? This is, however, a largely hypothetical question, because across geographically defined populations, there can be significant differences in morbidity, in the costs of access to health care and in the availability of resources (including the distribution of physicians), which means that different physicians see different kinds of patients and have different resources at their disposal. It is these differences which would commonly be seen as inequitable and of concern to governments which are aiming to promote equity in health care.

Medical practice variation may be defined in two ways. First, cross-sectionally, i.e. over the same period of time, differences will be observed in, e.g., the rates at which a geographically defined population receives treatment for a particular condition, or the way physicians treat cases as inpatients or as day patients or outpatients. Second, as a result of policy changes, physicians will vary their practice so that, e.g., the same physician will increase the rate of treatment of a particular condition or increase the proportion of cases treated as day cases.

These preliminary observations ought to suffice to show the potential conflict between governments' aiming for equity in health care and medical practice variation which results from physicians' seeking freedom to practise where and how they choose. Certainly, many governments would claim to have sought to pursue greater equity in health care. It is almost a definition of a civilised society that lack of *ability* to pay for health care is not a barrier to treatment. Indeed, it can be readily argued that this commitment to equity is the primary determinant of governments' willingness to finance health care. Perhaps as a consequence of governments' concern with containing costs, they also focus on the distribution of resources for health care. Distributional questions are of less concern to physicians. What matters for the physician is how to treat a sick individual in ways valued most by that individual with regard to both the means of treatment available and the likely outcomes. Yet physicians can be crucial in influencing the use of resources. This was one version of Roemer's law (Roemer, 1961) – that whatever the number of hospital beds available, they will be filled – is misplaced in focusing on hospital beds alone: the USA, with the reduction in the use of existing beds, provides ample evidence now to refute the 'law' that there is no such thing as an empty bed. The geographical distribution of physicians varies considerably. It is difficult to see how this can result in a situation which is equitable for patients living in different areas of a country, since access costs are then bound to vary.

The issue of equity as it presents itself to governments is important; to physicians, however, it is largely irrelevant. (Of course, they may choose to devote more of their time to the poor than to the rich because the former are in greater need – but that is presumably grounds of the *efficient* use of their time.) Thus, it is almost inevitable that leaving physicians discretion to practise largely where and how they choose will result in a situation where a patient presenting in different parts of a country will receive different care. Even if the availability of physicians is the same, medical practice variation may result in inequity because of variations in how the equitably distributed physicians practise.

Policy in the UK with respect to equity in health care is a particularly interesting example of relevance of medical practice variation to policies to promote equity. Analyses of such variations began in the UK 50 years ago with Glover's study of geographical variations in tonsillectomy rates (see Ham, 1988). Certainly there is consistent evidence relating geographical variations in utilisation of medical care to variations in supply. Since the Report of the Resource Allocation Working Party (RAWP:

Department of Health and Social Security, 1976), UK policy has claimed to be using methods which equalise the opportunity of access to health care for equal need. Thus, this policy is aimed at reducing medical practice variation. Within the context of geographical equity, however, it is clear that a RAWP-type policy will not *eliminate* medical practice variation.

More recently, the USA has sought to introduce a system of payment for hospitals aimed largely at containing costs – the Prospective Payment System (PPS) by Diagnosis-Related Group (DRG) for Medicare Patients, which has attracted considerable interest in other countries (Bardsley *et al.*, 1987). This system, while not couched in terms of resident populations geographically, has important implications for equity. It entails a reduction in medical practice variation in the use made of hospital resources for each admission by DRG.

While RAWP methods and PPS focus on the inputs to health care, there is a need for concern about the relationship of medical practice variation to outcomes. Deaths from certain diseases within specified age groups ought to be largely avoidable, given modern medical practice, and yet disturbingly wide variations have been reported in 'avoidable deaths' for European Community countries (Holland, 1988). In the context of efficiency, too, it is natural to seek to relate inputs to benefits and to allocate resources to maximise outcomes for a given total of resources. This concern underlies the advocacy of the use of estimates of costs per Quality-adjusted Life Year (Qaly) gained for determining priorities for different types of medical care (Williams, 1985). Output and efficiency concerns of medical practice variation are dealt with elsewhere in this volume. They are, however, clearly relevant to this chapter's focus on equity (as is discussed later).

In examining equity in health care, it becomes important to understand which kind of equity is being sought and why. This introduction has suggested that equity in health care and its relationship to medical practice variation are important. The existence of medical practice variation can create problems for governments seeking to promote equity in health care. Certainly there has to be *some* process of rationing in health care and, given the focus of their discipline, this is a natural subject of study for economists. However, equity poses serious problems for conventional economics because such economics is based on individuals' maximising their self-interest (McGuire *et al.*, 1988).

Bringing medical practice variations together with concerns for equity forces consideration of what the focus of policies for equity is and what it should be. For example, providing equal access to health care may be thought equitable, but if, when patients get there, doctors do different things, is *that* equitable?

Thus, this chapter attempts to do three things. First, it considers why it is that equity is important in health care. Second, it examines various possible definitions of equity and how such definitions are affected by the existence of medical practice variations. Third, it looks at policies to promote equity and the extent to which these are influenced by or take account of all the implications of medical practice variations.

WHY EQUITY IN HEALTH CARE?

Some Suggestions

The question of equity in health care appears to be important in that, in some form or other, it is a policy objective of most health care systems. It is then relevant to ask: why?

McGuire *et al.* (1988) have reviewed various possible justifications for equity in health care. This review reveals the difficulty the concept has created for economists as a subject of study. Thus, McGuire *et al.* wonder whether equity in health care is a legitimate interest for economists, and refer to Collard's observation (Collard, 1986) that self-interested economic man dominates economics textbooks, and rationality and self-interest are often taken as one and the same thing. Why, therefore, should individuals, normally expected to pursue their own selfish interests, be prepared to commit resources to be spent on the health care of others? This is a complex question, to which there are at least two answers, each of which is potentially relevant to the bases of health care policy.

One answer is that individuals gain utility from the welfare of others. This may take various forms. There may be some concern to avoid being affronted by the idea that people could die on the steps of a hospital when their lives would be saved if they were to be admitted. Or there may be a desire to provide 'adequate' health care for all. Again, the utility gained from others' welfare may be very broad, involving the notion of a better society which is caring in this way. McGuire *et al.* suggest that the concept proposed by Margolis of individuals possessing two utility functions may be the most useful basis for understanding equity (Margolis, 1982). One of these functions includes both the 'conventional' selfish function, and one which reflects utility derived from participating in attempting to produce benefits for some wider society. Each individual will have views on how marginal changes in his/her own resources should be allocated between society and the individual.

The second answer is that the altruistic basis of health care maximises self-interest even when it is defined narrowly. Thus, Titmuss (1973) argued that blood transfusion services were better organised on an altruistic rather than on a commercial basis. He used this as a particular example of the advantages of altruism, such as those that flow from a system of health care which is free at the point of consumption. This has emerged as a key issue with the risk of AIDS (and in the UK people have been infected with the virus through use of imported blood: Owen, 1988). As an additional point, Evans (1987) has recently argued that universal coverage which aims to secure equity turns out to be the most effective means of containing costs of health care. In contrast to Canada, the USA has problems both from the uninsured and from the escalating costs of health care for those who do have cover.

Consistency and Change over Time

McLachlan and Maynard (1982) drew attention to the surprising consistency in the definition of equity as a goal for health care between that of the UK wartime (1939–45) Coalition Government and those in statements by President Nixon in his message to Congress in 1972, and from Mrs Thatcher in a speech to the 1982 Conservative Party Conference, which was reiterated in the 1983 election manifesto (Maynard, 1987).

The UK Government's statement in 1944 set out its objective for health care as follows: 'the Government ... want to ensure that in the future every man and woman and child can rely on getting ... the best medical and other facilities available; and that their getting them shall not depend on whether they can pay for them or on any other factor irrelevant to real need' (Ministry of Health, *The National Health Service: A Summary of the Proposed Services*, Cmnd 6761, HMSO, 1946).

President Nixon described a national health strategy which aimed to give the whole population access to the best medical care and end any 'racial, economic or social barriers which prevent adequate health protection'. Mrs Thatcher stated: 'The principle that adequate health care should be provided for all regardless of ability to pay must be a foundation of any arrangements for financing health care.'

Although McLachlan and Maynard are correct in identifying consistency in stating equity as an objective for health care, they fail to point out the important shifts in emphasis which have occurred over how equity is defined. In the UK, in the 1940s, statements about equity in health care prior to the creation of the National Health Service were concerned with achieving the *best* medical care for all. The concerns of both President Nixon and Mrs Thatcher were about the removal of barriers to *adequate* health care.

This shift in definition is important for two reasons. First, it points to different underlying rationales about equity in medical care: is access to health care defined as a right in society, or is health care regarded as a 'merit good'? (i.e. a commodity which will be underconsumed if left to the willingness to pay of individual sovereign consumers, and is one for which some élite decides what the level of consumption ought to be)? Second, it raises important questions about how either definition is to be implemented and about how they differ given medical practice variation which results in both lack of clarity and lack of agreement in defining what is 'best' and what is 'adequate'. For example, what some physicians regarded as the 'best' may be regarded as only 'adequate' by others. Thus, Aaron and Schwartz (1984) suggest that UK physicians accept rationing which their counterparts in the USA would not.

Equity and Variation

It is possible to consider further reasons why equity in health care seems to matter and how such concerns, be they related to best or adequate care, have changed over time. Such considerations matter if we are to understand what the driving force behind equity is and ought to be attached to it. For example, if a society gains satisfaction from seeing itself as a fair, caring society, then such a society loses something if medical practice variations exist which result in much higher rates for some common procedure (such as hysterectomy) in one region than another. Is it possible to see this as fair, just or equitable? Again, if individuals want to do 'their fair share for society' (seeking utility from acting in this way, as Margolis suggested), they may be inhibited from contributing to this 'common good' if there is little in common in the way comparable patients are treated in different parts of the country (for example, lithotripsy and percutaneous surgery for removal of kidney stones).

For these reasons, equity and medical practice variation make unhappy bedfellows.

DEFINING EQUITY FOR HEALTH CARE POLICY

Consensus and Confusion

Equity is often seen as being essential in framing policies for health care: 'The stress of "Health for All" is on the last two words – the message of equity' (Abel-Smith, 1985). Consensus over the importance of equity in health care, however, is not matched by clarity over its definition (Mooney, 1983, 1987). For example, while the plan of action for the implementation of regional strategies of health for all of the Pan American Health Organisation (PAHO) identified equity as an essential attribute of health services. Musgrove (1986) notes that PAHO had not developed any way of monitoring progress towards equity. Again, Waddington and Newell (1987) report that the WHO Regional Office for the Western Pacific asked its 32 member states, as one of its indicators on progress towards the strategy of 'Health for All by the year 2000', whether resources were equitably distributed. Twenty said that they did not know, four said no and only eight claimed that their health resources were distributed equitably. As Waddington and Newell point out, this response, although worrying, is hardly surprising, as equity was not defined in the question. Mooney (1987) identified three different interpretations of equity by WHO in the Global and European strategies towards 'Health for All': equal health; reducing inequalities in health; and equity of access to primary health care.

Differing Definitions of Equity as Bases for Policies

Even when equity is clearly defined as an objective of policy, there is still scope for confusion in that the means chosen to pursue it may result in equity being achieved – but under a different definition. The creation of the UK National Health Service (NHS) in 1948 did not lead to equity in terms of access, as was intended, because the abandonment of price as a barrier to access removed only one (albeit an important one) of the possible barriers: other barriers remained, including certain features associated with social class and distance from services. Thus, although health services were largely 'free' at the point of consumption, nearly 30 years elapsed before RAWP was established to try to secure equal opportunity of access for equal need geographically. However, what its methods can achieve is more limited: the equalisation of resource use per capita adjusted for the estimated relative risk for health services but restricted to considerations of only hospital and community health services (Mooney, 1986). It is not simply that there is displacement from the stated objective of equalising opportunity of access. The approach adopted excludes primary care. Further, if RAWP's stated objective (i.e. equal opportunity of access for equal need) were to be achieved, it would require allowance for variations in the distribution of private health care and other social services, either of which may act as partial substitutes for public health services. Adjustment would also be needed to allow for variations in access which occur even when resources are equitably distributed – e.g. because of sparsity/density of the distribution of populations.

Types of Equity

Given the importance of equity in policies for health care, and confusion over what equity might mean, it is necessary to consider different ways of defining equity as a policy objective. Discussion of this issue provides the basis for examining the two questions of central concern: to what extent does variability in medical practice result in inequity in health care? and what assumptions are made about this variability in policies intended to promote equity?

Mooney (1983) has identified seven possible definitions of equity in terms of equality of: (1) expenditure per capita; (2) inputs per capita; (3) inputs for equal need; (4) utilisation for equal need; (5) access for equal need; (6) health; and (7) marginal met need. These are largely self-explanatory, except perhaps for the last – marginal met need. This approach assumes that if equity is sought geographically across different regions, then it is achieved when the 'marginal met need', i.e. that need which it is just possible to meet within the available resources, is the same. It requires a number of assumptions to apply this concept (see Steele, 1981), the most important of which is that each region ranks its priorities for meeting needs according to the benefit:cost ratio of doing so. In other words, that those who decide who gets treated aim to maximise the benefits from the available resources.

The above list is not exhaustive, but it covers some important ways in which equity may be defined and in which variation may occur. Each definition of equity is a ratio. The primary concern of the different definitions is in terms of the numerator – the only difference in the denominator lies in whether it is defined in terms of per capita or takes account of differences in the need for care.

What is the impact of medical practice variation on these different definitions? Three important points are worth making here.

First, none of the definitions *explicitly* incorporates the question of equitable deployment of physicians. Although those definitions concerned with the distribution of resources are clearly capable of doing so, as indicated below, simply allocating resources generally or expenditure equitably will not necessarily lead to equity in the distribution of physicians.

Second, variation in the distribution of physicians and other resources is likely to contribute to variations in medical practice which result in variations in assessments of needs, both quantitatively and qualitatively. Thus, it is postulated that as the costs to individuals of access increase, fewer people use the service, and that, *ceteris paribus*, the marginal benefit from treatment diminishes as more people get treated. In catchment populations where there are more physicians per capita (taking account of risk), the costs of access to care will be lower and a higher proportion of the population will be examined, there is likely to be a higher assessment of the need for health care with the marginal need met being lower. Even if physicians were distributed equitably, variations in the availability of equipment, technology and support staff may cause them to practise inequitably, i.e. physicians seeing the same kinds of patients will define their needs for health care differently.

Third, particularly for those definitions concerned with access and utilisation, even if the distribution of physicians is equitable and they agree on how need for health care is defined, variations in medical practice may still result in inequity. The point is a simple one. If patients have equal access to an equal utilisation of health care, if, when they get to the services, physicians then do different things, is this equitable?

It can, of course, be argued that these points can be incorporated into the definitions of equity listed above. That is not disputed. The issue is rather that in considering the equity implications of medical practice variations, one is forced to recognise not just the *quantitative* considerations incorporated into most definitions (and consequently formulae) of equity, but also the key role of the physician in how resources are in practice used, in how patients' needs are defined and in how the uncertainty associated with medical practice results in comparable patients receiving different treatment. This suggests that any definition of equity needs to accept the desirability of incorporating the concept of 'like' treatment for like needs, or the notion that individuals with similar problems have, for example, not only equal access to health care, but also equal opportunity to receive the same treatment.

Measuring Inequality

The first four types of equity defined above are all ratios of supply of health care to populations which can be defined by place of residence, social class or place of treatment. The definitions may differ because:

(1) Variations in price cause expenditure per capita to be different from inputs per capita.

(2) Variations in need cause inputs per capita to be different from inputs for equal need.

(3) Variations in medical practice cause inputs for equal need to be different from utilisation for equal need.

The remaining three definitions are concerned with different concepts from the first four and from each other: equity in access can only apply to populations of potential consumers of care; equity in outcome applies to populations of actual consumers who are supplied with care; marginal met need applies only to populations defined locationally. Differences between these definitions arise from:

(4) Variations in their costs of access.

(5) Variations in the cost-effectiveness of health care. Thus, equalising health outcomes will differ from equalising supply, and each will differ from equalising the ratio of marginal benefit of medical care to its marginal cost.

Medical practice variations cause serious problems in *measuring* inequity and in distinguishing between the different types.

A system of allocating resources which fails to take account of variations in price will result in physicians having an inequitable distribution of resources and therefore result in variation in medical practice. There are problems in accounting for variations in price for two reasons. First, where, as in the UK, the state approaches being a monopoly employer of health care professionals. For other groups of personnel it is possible to identify market variations in price but this does not apply to health care professionals. Standardisation of pay geographically will lead to problems in recruitment and retention which may lead to staff shortages. But to identify staff shortages ideally means that it is possible to relate staff to the need for them. Thus, to estimate the impact of variations in price or lack of variations in price it is necessary to have a measure of need for care. But this leads to a second problem if, as in the UK, equity is defined by resident populations but staff shortages are defined in terms of place of treatment: a resident population may be using resources at an inequitably high level and be treated in a hospital which is short of staff, given the cases being treated.

A major problem in measuring need for health care is that the existence of medical practice variation means that there is consistency neither in defining people in need nor in deciding on care to be provided for those deemed to be in need. This is illustrated by UK attempts to base measurement of need on populations by place of residence and US attempts to measure need by place of treatment.

In the UK resources are allocated on the basis of resident populations adjusted for the estimated need for health care. The problem in doing so is that ideally to measure need requires data on the underlying morbidity of different populations but no adequate data are available. Thus, it is necessary to find a suitable proxy. The data routinely collected by health services are of utilisation but unfortunately these data are unsatisfactory as a proxy for need, because use of health care is influenced by supply (Morgan *et al.*, 1987). Data are available on the age and sex distributions of populations and their mortality: these are direct indicators of need which are largely independent of supply. However, there are problems in deciding what relative weight to give to these different factors. The RAWP report (Department of Health and Social Security, 1976) recommended weighting the age/sex composition of regional populations by national average utilisation rates by age and sex, and multiplying these rates by their Standardised Mortality Ratios (SMRs). This recommendation is open to challenge, because actual national utilisation by age and sex may not reflect need for care (there may, for example, be more inadequate services for the elderly than for other groups) and there is no way of knowing whether the choice of a one-to-one weighting for SMRs is correct. Despite RAWP's rejection of relying on utilisation data as an indicator of need for health care, the recent review of the RAWP formula by the NHS Management Board (Department of Health and Social Security, 1988) has used such data as the basis for recommended changes in the formula: incorporating a weighting for an indicator of social deprivation (the Under-Privileged Area score) and reducing the weighting for SMRs to 0.44.

The USA has developed a system of paying hospitals according to the estimated needs of inpatients admitted, based on the DRG to which each patient has been assigned. There are nearly 500 DRGs, divided into medical and surgical groups: medical DRGs are generated by principal diagnosis; surgical DRGs by operating procedures. Some DRGs are further divided according to age, complications and comorbidities. Special provision is made for 'outliers', i.e. cases with stays or resource use significantly greater than the mean for their DRG. However, it is doubtful whether DRGs measure need for health care even in relative terms (Coffey and Goldfarb, 1986; Worthman and Cretin, 1986; Jencks and Dobson, 1987). PPS is essentially based on an estimate of average resource use from characteristics which are recorded in discharge abstracts. Thus, payment is calculated on what is done on average rather than what ought to be done or what is done in a particular instance. Practice within the hospital is subject to scrutiny by Peer Review Organisations, but, given medical practice variation, it is unclear how effective these can be in requiring only needed care to be provided. What is deemed to be needed will often vary between physicians without any clear prescription being available to enable such differences to be understood or, thereafter, resolved.

Variations in the costs of access to medical care and in the value different patients attach to it mean that physicians see only a self-selected sample. The existence of the clinical iceberg has been consistently documented. Policies which change access costs will then alter the populations which present to physicians. Medical practice will thus vary according to policies which influence access to medical care and consequently to access itself.

Variations in cost-effectiveness arise not only from differences in choice of therapy, but also from the management of any chosen therapy in terms of costs and outcomes. Physicians are restricted by what is available. Consequently, variations in the supply of resources are one factor in explaining medical practice variation. Beyond that, however, physicians with the same available supply will tend to differ in their choice and management of therapy.

POLICIES TO PROMOTE EQUITY: IMPLICATIONS FOR MEDICAL DISCRETION

Introduction

Although physicians perform a crucial role in translating symptoms presented by patients into demands for health care, they cannot frame these demands without a patient, nor can they guarantee that the demands they do frame will be met. They obviously have to take account of what is available. The question pursued here is that of how different policies to promote equity impinge on medical practice variation and alter the scope for medical discretion, which includes choice over *where* and *how* to practise medicine.

The argument that follows begins with the apparently easiest way of implementing a policy for equity: that followed by the USA, where cover is categorical and the focus for the system of payment is hospitals. It is suggested that the attempt to contain costs by PPS by DRG will fail because of medical practice variation and that a more effective approach is finance on a capitation basis. UK experience with this latter approach is then discussed by focusing on problems caused by medical practice variation. It is then argued that for the UK effective policies for equity in health care entail altering the geographical distribution of physicians (although it is accepted that even if there were equal distributions of physicians, variation would remain). The final question examined is the relevance of the concept of marginal met need to future policies for health care.

Equity by Need for Populations Treated in Hospitals

There have been two concerns about the US PPS by DRG: could DRGs provide an equitable basis for paying hospitals? and would PPS contain health care costs? Although debate continues over the first, essentially there is, in the USA, no real alternative to DRGs. The fundamental issue underlying the second question is whether the model of PPS by DRG can contain health care costs, given physicians' scope for manoeuvre allowed because of variation in medical practice. Wennberg *et al.* (1984) expected PPS by DRG to fail to contain the total costs of Medicare because of such variation. And indeed they were correct, but were wrong in predicting exactly how PPS would fail in this respect.

Wennberg *et al.* (1984) observed massive variation in admission rates by DRG, and predicted that the introduction of PPS would lead to empty beds through reductions in lengths of hospital stays, which could then be filled by physicians' increasing their rates of admissions. In the event, however, admission rates fell following the introduction of PPS (Schramm and Gabel, 1988).

It has been alleged that the decline in admission rates followed from the scrutinising by Peer Review Organisations of admissions (Schramm and Gabel, 1988). But PPS only constrained care provided to inpatients and did not apply to ambulatory care or fees to physicians. It was therefore to be expected that physicians would alter their practice away from inpatient care. This is exactly what has happened; although PPS is bringing some control to costs of inpatient care, there has been an explosion in the costs of ambulatory care, services provided in physicians' offices and fees to physicians (Iglehart, 1988; Schramm and Gabel, 1988). Thus PPS has failed to contain health care costs, as a result of medical practice variation.

As PPS has failed to contain costs of Medicare, there are essentially two options open to the US Federal Government: either to develop systems of measuring and controlling ambulatory care and physicians' services in ways analogous to DRGs, or to introduce a system of finance by capitation. The first entails measuring and regulating activity on a massive scale but, given medical practice variation, it is unclear how effective regulation would be. It is, therefore, not surprising that the administrator of the Health Care Financing Administration has advocated moving towards a system of finance by capitation (Iglehart, 1988).

Equity by Need by Residential Population

Current UK policy may be seen as a product of the characteristics of UK health care: since 1948 central government has had largely a monopoly

of finance and delivery; since 1974 responsibility for delivery is organised by health authorities defined geographically by resident populations; since 1976 the total finance for these authorities has been
cash-limited, determined prospectively. Given these characteristics, it is
natural to use a population-based formula to guide how the total should
be distributed to health authorities. Since 1976 the approach recommended by the Resource Allocation Working Party (RAWP) has been
used as a basis for such formulae in resource allocation, and this
approach has been followed in other countries in Scandinavia and
Australasia. The formula for revenue allocations estimates an equitable
distribution of resources (the 'target') which is typically different from
the existing allocation.

The applications of RAWP principles led to a need to reduce total
spending in inner London and ten-year strategies to achieve this by a
planned reduction in inpatient beds for acute inpatient care. (There was,
however, no explicit planned reduction in physicians.) The consequence
was a reduction in length of stay, and a massive increase in ambulatory
care. This has meant that the planned reductions in cost failed to
materialise: in the first two years of the ten-year strategy, three-quarters
of the planned reduction in beds had been implemented but only a third
of the planned savings had been achieved (King's Fund, 1987) –
although this may be partly explained by marginal cost lying below the
average.

What is of particular interest here is how very different policies
pursued in the USA and the UK have had similar consequences arising
from unpredicted variations in medical practice. The USA sought to
contain costs per inpatient admission – and succeeded, but at the same
time provided financial incentives for increases in other types of care,
which resulted in a failure to contain total costs. In the UK the attempt to
reduce costs by removing beds also resulted in reductions in lengths of
stay, but led to an explosion in ambulatory care and a failure to contain
costs. That these very different approaches produced similar results
shows the problems of supplier-induced demand where the key supplier is the physician. Evans (1987) makes a similar point about Canada,
where an increase in the numbers of physicians did not lead to
competition but to greater use of physicians' services. Klein (1975) was
perceptive in anticipating that to be effective a more equitable distribution of resources in the UK required a more equitable distribution of
physicians. He further suggested that the former would be easier to
achieve than the latter, as illustrated by the experience of attempting to
alter the geographical distribution of general practitioners in the UK
(Butler *et al.*, 1973).

For the UK Government, future policy options involve decisions
about total spending on hospital and community health services and

distributions of financial resources and physicians. There are broadly four unpalatable options from different mixes of these ingredients. These are:

(1) To continue with current policies: limited growth in total financial resources which are distributed equitably without altering the distribution of physicians.

(2) To continue with current policies of limited growth in total financial resources which are distributed equitably and move physicians out of London.

(3) To continue with the existing policy of achieving geographically equity but increase total allocations so that reductions are not required in London.

(4) To continue with current policies of limited growth in total financial resources, but not to alter the distribution of physicians and abandon the policy of distributing resources equitably.

Adequate Health Care for All?

The final point to consider brings together concerns about cost and outcome which underlie the concept of equity in terms of marginal met need. This is relevant to both the USA and the UK in their search for adequate health care for all. It might seem odd that the USA and the UK have a common problem here, given the different ideologies which underlie the provision of health care in each country (Culyer *et al.*, 1981). Consider, however, how the different systems work in practice.

In the UK everyone is supposed to have equal access to public health care. Those who buy private care do so on grounds of comfort, convenience and *not having to wait*. In the NHS there is believed to be no waiting for emergency admissions, but for 'cold' surgery people may have to wait a long time. Indeed they may die before they are treated. In the USA the Federal Government finances the costs of Medicare, which is such an important source of revenue that hospitals will want to be eligible for these revenues. To be eligible for Medicare income, hospitals have to accept all emergency cases whether the patients involved have cover or not. If they fail to accept an emergency case, they may lose their eligibility for Medicare. (This probably explains why PPS has not resulted in the 'dumping' of patients.) Thus, the relevant difference here between the countries is that whereas in the UK everyone is eligible for 'cold' surgery, but to be sure of getting it without too great a delay, you might have to make private arrangements; in the US eligibility for 'cold' surgery is restricted to those covered by the various private and public schemes.

A key issue here lies in the common acceptance that there should be no rationing of emergency care. One of the problems with this is that there is no consistent definition of what constitutes an 'emergency', and that this in itself can be an important source of variation. An interesting finding of the research stimulated by the introduction of PPS by DRG was that there was more variation in rates of admission for medical DRGs than surgical DRGs (Wennberg *et al.*, 1984; Lagoe, 1986). It is also relevant to ask what benefits come from emergency admissions. If the concern is to ration resources effectively, then it is essential to review both the outcomes resulting from the convention which gives priority to emergency admissions and variations in how 'emergencies' are defined.

CONCLUSION

This chapter has sought to explore some of the relationships between medical practice variation and inequity in health care and has aimed to establish two main points: first, that variations in the distribution of physicians will result in variations in medical practice; and second, that variations in medical practice, in the sense of doctors' doing different things to comparable patients – often with unknown impact on health – makes it difficult to provide satisfactory ways of measuring inequity. This means that any government which aims to secure a more equitable distribution of health care confronts a potentially vicious circle: to alter the distribution of physicians requires a strong argument based on measures of inequity, while at the same time the existing distribution results in variation in medical practice which means that any measure of need for health care is contentious. But, as the costs of medical care are most effectively contained through a system of capitation-based finance, governments have to confront this vicious circle.

The problem governments face is how to move towards a system of rationing health care *both* equitably and efficiently. To do so, it is necessary to develop a policy based on three elements. First, there is the necessity to use crude measures of need to determine the degree of inequity that exists within a country. Typically, the degree of inequity discovered far exceeds the errors likely from the use of crude measures; second, to use those crude measures to equalise the distribution of total resources; and third, to consider the cost-effectiveness of the mix within those totals.

Medical practice variation arises partially – but only partially – from differences in the number and type of physicians in each area and the resources available to them. Equalising total resources without altering the distribution of physicians will create problems of frustration in areas losing resources and lack of effective use of the increased resources distributed to other areas. The mix of physicians will largely determine the health care provided: increasing the ratio of medical specialists will increase emergency care; increasing the ratio of surgeons will increase scope for cold surgery. The health care provided will also obviously be a product of other resources for diagnosis and treatment.

Thus, the policy outlined here does not entail case-by-case scrutiny of medical practice in an attempt to get to grips with medical practice variations. In that respect it is appealing to physicians. In other respects it implies considerable constraints on physicians' choices over the type of medicine and the place in which they will practise. Such a policy encounters difficulties in terms of acceptability to physicians or knowledge about health care. For example, it suggests influencing choices at a formative stage of physicians' careers, with uncertainty at that time as to what kinds of medicine will be most cost-effective when they are fully trained. Given these implications of the impact of equity on variations in medical practice, it is hardly surprising that, although there is consensus between governments about the desirability of equity in health care, this consensus is marked by confusion. For this reason, it will be surprising if the future results in any greater clarity in government policies for equity in health care.

It is hoped, however, that this chapter has made clear that, given medical practice variation, pursuing policies on equity which are based solely on manipulating the distribution of resources in general is unlikely to be successful on its own. The key resource – physicians – needs special attention to reduce the impact of medical practice variation on inequities in services actually delivered. It is also necessary to understand the degree to which medical practice variation would result from medical discretion, even given an equitable distribution of physicians and other health care resources. If this would indeed result in substantial inequities in service delivery, then this would pose challenges to medical education, medical practice and medical knowledge. The nature of these challenges has been described in other chapters. This chapter has shown their potential relevance to the pursuit of equity in health care.

REFERENCES

Aaron, H. J. and Schwartz, W. B. (1984). *The Painful Prescription*. The Brookings Institution, Washington, D.C.

Abel-Smith, B. (1985). Global perspectives on health service financing. *Soc. Sci. Med.*, **20**, 957–63

Bardsley, M., Coles, J. and Jenkins, L. (Eds.) (1987). *DRGs and Health Care: the Management of Case Mix*. King Edward's Hospital Fund, London

Butler, J. R., Bevan, J. M. and Taylor, R. C. (1973). *Family Doctors and Public Policy*. Routledge and Kegan Paul, London

Coffey, R. M. and Goldfarb, M. G. (1986). DRGs and disease staging for reimbursing medicare patients. *Med. Care*, **24**, 814–29

Collard, D. (1986). *Altruism and Economy: A Study in Non-selfish Economics*. Martin Robertson, Oxford

Culyer, A. J., Maynard, A. and Williams, A. (1981). Alternative systems of health care provision: an essay on motes and beams. In Olson, M. (Ed.), *A New Approach to the Economics of Medical Care*. American Enterprise Institute, Washington, D.C.

Department of Health and Social Security (1976). *Sharing Resources for Health in England. Report of the Resource Allocation Working Party* (The RAWP Report). HMSO, London

Department of Health and Social Security (1988). *Review of the Resource Allocation Working Party Formula. Final Report by the NHS Management Board*. DHSS, London

Evans, R. G. (1987). Public purchase of health insurance: the collective provision of individual care. *Hlth Policy*, **7**, 115–34

Ham, C. (Ed.) (1988). *Health Care Variations*. King's Fund, London

Holland, W. W. (1988). *European Community Atlas of Avoidable Death*. Oxford University Press, Oxford

Iglehart, J. K. (1988). Payment of physicians under Medicare. *New Engl. J. Med.*, **318**, 863–8

Jencks, S. F. and Dobson, A. D. (1987). Refining case-mix adjustment. *New Engl. J. Med.*, **317**, 679–86

King's Fund (1987). *Planned Health Services for Inner London*. King's Fund, London

Klein, R. (1975). The National Health Service. In Klein, R. (Ed.). *Inflation and Priorities: Social Policy and Public Expenditure, 1975*. Centre for Studies in Social Policy, London, pp. 83–104

Lagoe, R. L. (1986). Differences in hospital discharge rates. *Med. Care*, **24**, 868–72

McGuire, A., Henderson, J. and Mooney, G. (1988). *The Economics of Health Care*. Routledge and Kegan Paul, London

McLachlan, G. and Maynard, A. (1982). The regulation of public and private markets. In *The Public/Private Mix for Health*. Nuffield Provincial Hospitals Trust, London, pp. 515–58

Margolis, H. (1982). *Selfishness, Altruism and Rationality*. Cambridge University Press, Cambridge

Maynard, A. (1987). Markets and health care. In Williams, A. (Ed.), *Health and Economics*. Macmillan, London, pp. 187–200

Ministry of Health (1946). *The National Health Service; A Summary of the Proposed Services* (Cmd 6761). HMSO, London

Mooney, G. (1983). Equity in health care: confronting the confusion. *Effective Hlth Care*, **1**, 179–84

Mooney, G. (1986). *Economics, Medicine and Health Care*. Wheatsheaf, Brighton

Mooney, G. (1987). What does equity in health mean? *Wld Hlth Stat. Q.*, **40**, **4**, 296–303

Morgan, M., Mays, N. and Holland, W. W. (1987). Can hospital use be a measure of need for health care? *J. Epidemiol. Commun. Hlth*, **41**, 269–74

Musgrove, P. (1986). Measurement of equity in health. *Wld Hlth Stat. Q.*, **39**, 325–35

Owen, D. (1988). *Our NHS*. Pan, London

Roemer, M. I. (1961). Bed supply and hospital utilisation: A natural experiment. *Hospitals*, 1 November, 35–42

Schramm, C. J. and Gabel, J. (1988). Prospective payment. Some retrospective observations. *New Engl. J. Med.*, **318**, 1681–6

Steele, R. (1981). Marginal unmet need and geographical equity in health care. *Scot. J. Pol. Econ.*, **28**, 186–95

Titmuss, R. (1973). *The Gift Relationship*. Penguin, Harmondsworth

Waddington, C. and Newall, K. (1987). Different therefore equal: towards equity in the health services in Fiji. *Asia-Pacific J. Publ. Hlth*, **1**, 24–31

Wennberg, J. E., McPherson, K. and Caper, P. (1984). Will payment based on Diagnosis-Related Groups control hospital costs? *New Engl. J. Med.*, **311**, 295–300

Williams, A. (1985). The economics of coronary artery bypass grafting. *Br. Med. J.*, **291**, 326–9

Worthman, L. G. and Cretin, S. (1986). *Review of the Literature of Diagnosis Related Groups*. A RAND Note, N-2492-HCFA. Santa Monica, Calif.

CHAPTER 6

Measuring Performance in the Health Care Sector: the Whys and the Hows

Alistair McGuire

INTRODUCTION

Over the recent past there has been a fundamental reassessment of the role of the public sector and the level of public expenditure in all the industrialised countries. To some extent this reassessment has been associated with – indeed has been a result of – the continued growth of public expenditure during the post-war period. Policy concerns are increasingly directed at the evaluation of the costs and benefits associated with the Welfare State. As importantly, however, this reassessment has occurred because the growth has been accompanied by a significant change in composition, largely away from expenditure on goods and services towards transfer payments. This change in composition has also reflected a move away from the provision of traditional public goods (e.g. defence) towards those associated with the growth of the Welfare State, which has provided benefits on an individualistic basis and where redistributive concerns are dominant.

It is, therefore, not surprising that there has been increasing attention paid to the economic evaluation of health care: it represents a significant redistributive content, and the benefits are largely, although not exclusively, individualistic. Recently particular interest has focused on efficiency in the health care sector. With this increased interest in efficiency, it has quickly become apparent that, because major resources decisions are taken by individual doctors who are not necessarily aware of the cost consequences, efficiency concerns must impinge on clinical decision making. This has in itself led to an increased questioning of the basis of such decision making and the accompanying outcomes. The now substantial evidence on medical practice variations has furthered such questioning. Inevitably attempts to control costs and to reduce practice variations have run into conflict with notions of clinical freedom. This chapter looks at some of the reasons why this conflict has arisen in the light of examining the use of efficiency measures in the UK.

Later the chapter examines some of the measures used in the UK to monitor performance. While these *are* UK-based the issues that emerge for further consideration are relevant to all health care systems. In particular, the question of how to define inefficiency in the health care sector, given the presence of extensive medical practice variation, is highlighted. As such, this chapter concentrates on the efficiency consequences of such variations and the measurement of associated inefficiency in the context of the performance of health care systems.

WHAT IS MEANT BY MEASURING EFFICIENCY?

The measurement of efficiency is one of the frequent tasks of the economist. Yet, as Hall and Whinston (1959) pointed out some time ago, the concept of efficiency is an ambiguous one. Efficiency may relate to the actual productive unit (an industrial plant, say) as judged *ceteris paribus* by its output levels. Alternatively, performance criteria may relate to managerial efficiency. If so, we would then have to take account of the environmental factors affecting managerial discretion – output levels alone would not suffice as performance indicators. Labour may be abundant in one part of the country but not in another; then, although two managers are involved in the production of exactly the same commodity, and may in fact produce the same output levels, they are operating under different conditions and this will affect judgement of their managerial performance. A further definition of efficiency relates to comparisons of a number of different production units operating with different techniques – process efficiency. Yet another aspect of efficiency may relate to organisational structure. It is important to recognise that the aspect of efficiency which is relevant will be dictated by the question being addressed. We may be concerned with relative output levels *per se*, relative constraints, relative techniques of production or organisational and managerial structure.

At its crudest and most general level, efficiency or performance relates to the degree of success in achieving stated objectives. This in itself does beg the question: 'what are the objectives?' Simple and straightforward as this question may seem, a common basic fault in the specification of performance indicators is the failure to make explicit and to justify the objectives being pursued. Of course, in making choices about competing objectives we are relying on value judgements concerning their relative worth. Once the objectives and value judgements implied by the adoption of various performance indicators are made explicit, the potentially contentious nature of the adopted indicators is fully revealed.

Unfortunately, little concern has in fact, in most countries, been given to the explicit specification of the objectives to be pursued by the health care sector. The usual response given to this criticism is to state that the objective is to provide the highest level of services that resources allow, or to maximise the benefit to society from health care services at least cost. This merely leads us back to definitional problems: what do we mean by maximum benefits or the highest level of services?

Of course, given this lack of concern with objectives, it is hardly surprising that there are substantial medical practice variations. If there is both a lack of discussion and a lack of agreement on objectives which might guide clinicians in their activities, there will almost inevitably be differences of opinion across clinicians in how to maximise benefit and how to provide the highest level of services.

In its report in 1979 the Royal Commission on the UK National Health Service (the NHS) listed five distinct objectives. These were: to encourage and assist individuals to remain healthy; to provide equality of entitlement to health care; to provide a broad range of services of high standard; to satisfy the reasonable expectations of users; and to remain a national health service free at the point of use.

It is possible to aggregate these objectives in different ways and to argue over the priorities to be given to each. Indeed it is instructive to repeat what the Royal Commission itself stated at the time (Cmnd. 7615):

'The absence of detailed and publicly declared principles and objectives for the NHS reflects to some degree the continuing political debate about the service. Politicians and public alike are agreed on the desirability of a national health service in broadly its present form, but agreement often stops there. Instead of principles there are policies which change according to the priorities of the day and the particular interests of the ministers concerned.'

Yet there are no correct number of objectives to be pursued or single ones which are naturally more important than others. The objectives and the importance to be attached to them will reflect the value judgements of the populace served. And just as these value judgements change over time, so will the objectives and the priorities. This is not to imply that explicit specification of objectives should not form the basis for policies, but rather that such objectives need not be static and unchanged. They are bound to change, to reflect the dynamic elements contained in attitudes and expectations.

Thus, the actual specification of the ruling objectives is a fundamentally difficult task. But this difficult and fundamental problem is normally overwhelmed by the immediacy of measurement problems – i.e. the question of how we measure the benefits or the level of provision of service replaces that of what we mean by benefit or level of provision. In other words, although we do not know what we are meant to be doing, let us measure what is actually going on in any case! And in fact, because this is in itself very difficult, we find that once time is allocated to this task there is little time left to consider what it is we ought to be doing.

WHY NOT LET THE MARKET DICTATE PERFORMANCE?

But why do we have to worry about monitoring performance? In other sectors of the economy, it is suggested that the market ensures that if a firm is not operating efficiently, it will quickly go out of business. Why is this not the case with health care? For a number of reasons markets can not provide health care efficiently. To see why this is the case, it is first of all worth noting that we are in fact normally considering two separate but interconnected commodities when we analyse the provision of health care; health care and health care insurance (see also Evans, 1984; McGuire *et al.*, 1988).

It is widely acknowledged that the market fails to provide either commodity efficiently. We shall consider the failures associated with each commodity in turn, starting with health care itself. Consumers of health care (patients) lack information about the timing of consumption needs; on the level and form of treatment required; and about the effectiveness of treatment. While a lack of information may affect the consumption of other commodities, its effect is particularly severe in the consumption of health care. A number of characteristics differentiate health care from other commodities. As with a number of goods and services, the consumer (in this case the patient) relies on the supplier (here the doctor) for information on product quality.

However, not only is it difficult for consumers of health care to judge quality before consumption, but also it is difficult for them to judge quality after consumption (Weisbrod, 1978). Patients rarely know whether the treatment was beneficial – they might have recovered in any case or they might have recovered more quickly with a different treatment. Moreover, because they do not (it is hoped) consume health care very often, they have little in the way of past experience to go on. And, of course, the costs of pursuing a wrong decision in health care are liable to be more severe and less reversible than in other areas of choice. Yet the costs of obtaining a second opinion (i.e. more information) are necessarily high, given the uncertainties involved. Notice, then, that the supplier of health care is providing two distinct services – information and treatments. The consumer (patient) relies on information from the supplier (doctor) concerning both the nature and the outcome of the consumption process and then for the provision of treatment itself. Notice also that the consumer derives satisfaction ('utility', in the jargon of the economist) from health *per se* and not from health care itself. This is important, as it emphasises that it is health outcome and not health care that should provide the basis for the evaluation of performance.

It will be recognised that supply decisions dominate this sector. The medical profession have a secure monopoly over the information necessary to define consumption – but this is not surprising, as this is, after all, why we train doctors. However, this monopoly operates at a very individual level. Therefore, the consumer may actually seek a second opinion from another member of the medical profession or, indeed, one doctor may challenge the diagnosis of another. Thus, the monopoly is over the information held by individual doctors and is merely subject to the regulation and approbation of the profession. Obviously, if left to the market, the monopoly potential of the supplier with regard to this information over product quality may be realised. Consumers have little knowledge of the product, so doctors could charge an excessive price for their services in the open market, as they also have a relatively secure monopoly over the provision of treatment.

To avoid any such realisation of monopoly advantage, the sector is regulated and the set of exchange relationships which normally char-acterises a market are replaced by various non-market relations (Arrow, 1963; Evans, 1981). Of particular importance is the agency relationship which exists between the doctor and the patient. Not only does the doctor act as a supplier of health care, but also he acts as an agent for the consumer (patient) in specifying the appropriate treatment pattern. This is one reason for the importance of medical ethics and conduct in the health care sector – it reassures the patient that the doctor is not exploiting his monopoly position with respect to information holdings in order to gain financially but is operating with the patient's best medical interests at heart. This may not always appear to be the case, but it does provide a normative rationale for the prominence of medical ethics in medicine. Of course, this separation of medical from economic concerns is aided by the third party payment system which is common to most developed health care systems – of which more below.

The inadequacies of the consumer's information and the potentially disastrous costs associated with making a wrong decision in consuming health care severely limit the consumer's choices. The doctor/supplier acts as an agent for the consumer and thereby can substantially affect the choices of the patient over consumption (i.e. treatments). Notice also that the monopoly over information held by the medical profession makes it difficult for the government to control directly the production of health care. It is partly for this reason that the medical profession holds substantial rights to self-government – i.e. it is largely left to the profession to control and monitor itself at the corporate level.

Yet it must be recognised that medical conduct, which dictates the nature of the production process, has little explicit concern with the resource implications (and therefore the costs) of that process. True, the individual doctor may be continually juggling his resources to meet the demands of his own patients, but there is little recognition of the real opportunity costs of the resources used (i.e. the alternative beneficial uses to which they could have been put). Not surprisingly, the self-regulation practised by the medical profession is aimed primarily at the profession's medical conduct rather than the economic implications of that conduct; it is aimed at regulating health care and not, for example, health care insurance.

In considering the economic or resource aspects of producing health care, we must consider this second commodity – health care insurance. The occurrence of illness is unpredictable. Individuals are uncertain about not only the timing of their future health care consumption, but also the form of that consumption and therefore also its cost. For this reason, they have recourse to insurance. Unfortunately, for reasons which are outlined briefly, the market fails to provide adequate insurance cover for health care. There are three main reasons for this failure.

First, insurance is really a matter of pooling risks. For insurance to be appropriate, the risk of the occurrence of the insurable event must be less than unity: i.e. the event must not be a certain occurrence. Just as it is not possible to insure your house if you knew that it would certainly be burgled or set on fire, it is not possible to gain insurance coverage if you are certain to need health care. The only way insurers could make a profit in such a situation would be to increase premiums by a substantial sum. Then it would not be worth while insuring. This immediately raises problems for those people with chronic illnesses, congenital problems and the older segments of society (i.e. the certainty of illness, and therefore the requirement for health care, increase with age).

Second, there is the problem of adverse selection, which arises when there is an asymmetry of information between the parties involved in the insurance contract. Individuals may have more information on their expected health status than the seller of insurance. Those who recognise that they face a high level of risk may deceive the insurance company and reap a financial reward in the form of a lower than actuarially fair insurance premium. This imposes costs on the insurance company and, if they can transmit these costs, on to other individuals seeking insurance. It may eventually lead to gaps in insurance coverage as insurers try to identify and then exclude high-risk individuals from coverage.

The third major problem is what is termed 'moral hazard'. Insured individuals have little incentive to restrict their consumption levels to those that would prevail if they faced the full cost of consumption. If medical insurance covers all costs, health care is effectively a free good to the consumer. Not surprisingly, there are fewer restrictions on the level of consumption in such circumstances than if the patient were faced with the full cost. Health insurers may attempt to exert some control by introducing co-insurance policies, but, given the high costs of a significant amount of health care, this, again, may lead to problems of exclusion.

In short, the market fails to provide an efficient means of providing health care coverage – either because of loadings on premiums and/or gaps in coverage. The most readily available evidence on this inefficiency is the estimated 12% of the US citizenry without health insurance coverage at any point in time. Indeed, it was the failure of the market to provide insurance that led to the introduction of the Medicare and Medicaid programmes in the USA in the mid-1960s.

REGULATING THE MARKET

It is against these market failures that the issues of regulation, and consequently the monitoring of performance, in the health care sector must be judged. Regulation applies to both the provision of health care and the provision of health care insurance. The regulatory regime imposed on one sector must be supportive of the other if these primary market failures in the provision of health care and health insurance are not to be replaced by even greater distortions. Thus, it should be continually emphasised that, for example, in the UK the NHS, while it arose largely for equity reasons, does have inherent regulatory characteristics particularly associated with the financing of and the provision of health care. The problems associated with health care insurance provision are overcome in the UK by financing health care from general taxation. The insurance solution does not work effectively and has been replaced by general taxation. There are no gaps in coverage and no administrative costs associated with the calculation and collection of insurance premiums. Indeed, 'insurance' is, technically, not the appropriate term to apply to a collective financing of the full range of costs that are incurred by individuals collectively. We may more appropriately term it 'the financing of health care through public finance'.

While this could lead to overconsumption, particularly as associated with the problem of moral hazard mentioned above, in aggregate this occurs less than might be expected, because the NHS is explicitly rationed through the public expenditure system. This rationing process is supported inasmuch as doctors receive a salary rather than payment on a fee-for-service basis, which also undermines any tendency towards oversupply. It is, after all, the doctors, acting on behalf of their patients, thereby overcoming the difficulties in the provision of health care stemming from consumer ignorance, who make the consumption choices. The major problems relating to efficiency and health care arise because consumers/patients do not have adequate information to make appropriate choices over their purchases of health care. Their doctor therefore acts as an agent on their behalf, and the medical conduct of individual doctors is regulated by the medical profession.

It will be appreciated, then, that the market (through the laws of supply and demand) does not operate efficiently in the health care sector for the reasons just outlined. However, abandoning a flawed (market) solution does not overcome all problems. The market is an efficient resource allocation mechanism because it can, under appropriate supporting conditions, effortlessly co-ordinate consumption and production activities by means of information conveyed by price signals. As we have seen, there are fundamental reasons why the market fails to undertake the allocation task efficiently in the health care sector. Obvious as it may be, it must be stressed that the market's failings and its replacement should be judged primarily on efficiency grounds and not solely on political or ideological grounds, if we are concerned with efficiency questions.

In the UK the health care market has been replaced by a planned system. Information transmission no longer has a price system to rely on – which is part of the reason why the monitoring of performance becomes so critical. (Not, of course, that pricing gets a free hand in other health care systems, such as in the US.) One of the main practices of the planning system must be to communicate to producers the values and output targets determined by the decision makers. As resources are controlled through the setting of expenditure levels or by some other method that puts a ceiling on the value of the inputs used in production, targets must be set in full recognition of the existing resource constraints, if they are to be realistic. In a system with vague objectives, uncertain outputs and in many cases unknown costs (as associated with resource use), it is not surprising that it is difficult to undertake any evaluation or regulation of performance. This is particularly true of a planned system, given that there are no self-adjusting mechanisms to correct false information flows. In a planned system information must be collected and collated before it can be assessed, whether or not the allocation is moving towards the target. Only after this has been done can the performance of the sector be assessed.

It is obvious to even those with limited knowledge of the sector that the existing planning system is itself not operating efficiently in the NHS. Not enough consideration has been given to the objectives to be pursued at an operational level; to what information is required to trace the movement towards such objectives; and to how resources should be allocated (on the basis of priority) between these objectives. It is true that resources are spent on collecting information (although, to keep this in perspective, the UK spends very little relatively on administration compared with other health care systems). However, until the objectives of the system are explicitly outlined, it is impossible to state whether such information is useful, let alone properly used.

WHY IS IT SO DIFFICULT TO IMPROVE PERFORMANCE IN A REGULATED SYSTEM?

To complicate matters further, there are definite measurement problems in the NHS. The actual health care production process is itself rather unique. By a production process is meant the transmission of inputs into outputs – in the health care sector we may think of the inputs as the labour (i.e. the doctors, nurses, etc.), drugs and capital that produce a 'treatment'. In other sectors of the economy this transmission of inputs into outputs is relatively straightforward. There is a recognised process that transforms inputs into outputs and the costs and processes involved are predictable across various volumes. In the health care sector this transformation of inputs into outputs is typically not pure. Not only can there be considerable scientific uncertainty concerning the effectiveness of treatment (i.e. the actual relationship between inputs and outputs), but also production is characterised by choices concerning the internal organisational and process aspects of treatment delivery. This means that actual organisation issues, involving when and how treatment is applied, as well as the representation and communication of diagnosis and treatment to the patient, are fundamental to the production of health care. Considerable discretion can be used over the choice of production process (Berki, 1983). Furthermore, any particular diagnostic problem may be approached and treated in a number of ways, in many cases with similar outputs. Alternatively, because of the intermediate nature of hospital production, exact similarity of treatment may result in a variety of outputs. In short, the efficiency of production processes is a function of the characteristics of the individual institutions and, indeed, the individuals within these institutions. Different indi-

viduals will have different perceptions of what constitutes good practice. This is the fundamental reason why medical practice variations
exist.

Given the nature of the product health care, it is not surprising to find
that these aspects are highly individualistic. As such as they are difficult
to regulate. This is not just because they are difficult to observe and
measure, but also because they may be particular to the individual
transaction – there is a tendency towards uniqueness in health care as
the complexity of the production process increases.

The uncertainty associated with the timing and form of health care
production has a number of impacts on the production process itself.
First, the process must be focused on short-term decision making and
resource allocation – in this sense it may be defined as a spot market
(any analogy with the financial market is deliberate, as it gives a good
impression of the intensity of resource allocation problems faced by
clinicians). Because health care is difficult to store, in that, being a
service, it is difficult to build up inventories, and it is produced and
delivered simultaneously on demand, decision making is geared to
immediate production problems. The decision-making process is characterised by adaptive, sequential pathways, while the production process (i.e. the diagnosis, information and, particularly, treatment) must
also be quickly responsive to changed requirements (Harris, 1977).

This makes the resource allocation problem and the associated
information flows extremely complex. Yet these aspects are critical to
the organisation of health care delivery: typically, successive adapta-
tions to changes in requirements arising from both the patient's health
and the constraints faced by the clinician are needed if efficient
production performance is to be realised. Moreover, the production
process deals with value added. Health care exists to contribute to
health status, but it is only one of many contributions. In this sense it
'adds value' to health status but does not produce health status *per se*.
Thus, while it is hoped but not necessarily so that improved health
status is the ultimate gain, value added is often calculated by focusing
on the services provided, the number of cases treated or the number of
successful cases, such measures implying that services are effective –
indeed, are of known effectiveness. Each outcome gives rise to different
specifications of the production process. Both clinical effectiveness and
economic efficiency must be assessed, bearing in mind the importance
of value added to the production process. It is no good focusing on the
level of services provided if no account is taken of the number of cases
treated or the number of successful cases. It is because final outcome can
vary so much in relation to the value added by health care that clinical
effectiveness is difficult to assess (see Chapter 3 in this volume).

In short, the health care sector is a complex array of individual, short-term decisions controlled largely by clinicians, operating as agents for patients. This agency role is subject to the self-regulatory mechanisms of the medical profession. Given the nature of the commodity and its production, this self-regulatory role is not straightforward. It is important to emphasise that this self-regulation focuses, quite legitimately, on medical conduct and not on economic conduct – except, of course, to the extent that economic conduct underlies medical conduct. However, this is not to say that medical doctors, either individually or as a profession, do not take decisions that have no economic consequences, but rather that their concern lies with the medical use to which these resources can be put, as opposed to the cost. Indeed, it is these economic consequences that are currently coming under increasing regulation.

In the UK it is widely believed that the NHS has been successful in synthesising the medical and the economic dimensions. The greater separation of financial determination from provision requirements which, to date at least, has been enjoyed by this publicly financed and provided system in relation to insurance-based systems, has, indeed, meant that there has been little reconciliation of medical conduct and resource allocation at the individual level. This has allowed the agency relationship to develop apparently unhindered by economic realities. However, as demands on the system have grown and as resource constraints have increasingly tightened, it is not surprising that greater attention has started to be paid to the economic consequences of medical conduct. While attention initially focused on the cost of services provided, it has already begun to move around to consideration of the associated treatment. The point is that consideration of production at one level (of value added) inevitably leads on to consideration at another level. In other words, given the inevitable connection between medical and economic activity at some level in the production process, it is also the case that examination of efficiency inevitably forces examination of effectiveness. In so far as medical practice variations – or at least certain aspects of them – are a symptom of inefficiency, then, as indicated elsewhere in this volume, examination of such variations necessitates an examination of effectiveness.

INDICATORS OF PERFORMANCE – BUT PERFORMANCE OF WHAT?

Ironically, the success achieved by the NHS, in divorcing medical decision making from its economic consequences, may account for the widespread belief that the overall performance has been good. If we cannot clearly discern what resources are going into any particular process and what resources can be attributed to any particular outcome, then, as long as, in aggregate, we are maintaining expenditure within the publicly determined amount and our crude morbidity and mortality figures are not grossly out of line with comparable countries, we must be performing relatively well. But this particular diagnosis misses the mass of cracks that closer inspection reveals, such as those revealed by the presence in the system of substantial variations across different geographical areas of medical practice. Such an aggregate view of performance does indeed highlight admirable grains of efficiency; in particular, the inefficiencies of the insurance market are replaced by the comprehensive coverage of public insurance, which has the added attraction of giving everyone financial equality of access to health care. This does considerably reduce administrative costs – but at the expense of not relating individual episodes of treatment to their resource cost.

It may be thought that by integrating public finance with provision, monitoring and control of resource usage would be easier than under a system where these functions were discrete. Certainly, the potential for such gains does exist, but until relatively recently this potential had not been realised in the UK – largely because the information on individual treatment costs has not been available. As a result, while the financing of the NHS has been strictly monitored through the public expenditure determination process, provision and resource usage, as determined by the individual clinician, has generally been haphazard and certainly unplanned. Resource allocation within the health care sector relies partly on a 'robbing Peter to pay Paul' approach, partly on a notion of historical precedence and partly on a principle of 'who shouts loudest, gets'. It is, therefore, not surprising that certain specialties have been seen to do better than others and that variation in how resources are used within each specialty remains.

One implication of the past blurring of medical and economic decision making is that clinicians, both individually and as a profession, have not perceived their domain as encompassing resource allocation procedures. Therefore, partly through default, attempts to reconcile these two aspects of health care decision making have tended to be derived from the aggregate level. Central government bodies – in particular, the Department of Health – have initiated measures for monitoring resource expenditure. Given the difficulties involved in defining and measuring clinical activity, it is not surprising that such measures have focused on the first stage of the value-added process – i.e. the reconciliation of expenditure with throughput levels, manpower levels, length of stay, and the like. Even so, the importance of attempting to use such measures should not be underestimated. They are at least an attempt, even if a rather poor one, to measure performance at a lower level of aggregation than has ever been attempted before. It is comparative performance that is being measured across the health sector nationally – an attempt to identify who is doing what and to whom. To do this successfully is a vital first step in the process of monitoring and controlling resource use in the sector. However, the question has to be posed whether performance indicators as have been developed to date, are 'successful'.

Important as such a move is, it is not without its own problems. While monitoring moves to a lower level than before, it remains above that which reconciles clinical activity with resource usage – which is, after all, what drives the system. It is not clear what focusing on an intermediate level will tell us. Given our discussion so far, it is not surprising that variation in medical outcomes exist. Such variation occurs not merely because of the individual characteristics associated with any one patient, but also because of the nature of the production process itself *and*, maybe most importantly, the individual characteristics of the doctor. What remains to be assessed is whether such variation is compatible with efficiency. Focusing attention on variations will not in itself reveal the cause of variation. It may relate to something about medical management, although even here we would have to be careful to control for differences in other resource levels.

UK performance indicators may be aggregated into five groups. These are clinical, financial, manpower, ambulance and estate management indicators. Clinical indicators, for example, include such measures as length of stay, admission rate, waiting lists per 1000 population, etc. It is enlightening to consider the official view concerning such attempts to measure performance:

'It is necessary at this stage to be clear what performance indicators are and what they are not. They are not and cannot be absolute measures of performance in terms of achieved health care. There must be ultimately a clinical measurement and we are a long way from getting into that territory. What they essentially comprise are rankings of all the 192 districts in the English health service in competitive order of performance against certain indicators' [Sir Kenneth Stowe, Permanent Secretary at the DHSS, on the introduction of performance indicators, cited in evidence to the Public Accounts Committee, 1983–84, p. 25].

From this statement it should be clear that performance indicators, as used in the UK, are not wholly concerned with measuring improvements in health status. Nor are they solely concerned with *medical* practice variation. Rather, they are measures of the throughput of resources, introduced as part of an overall tightening of the monitoring and control system of the NHS with the general objective of constraining public expenditure levels. The objective of restraining growth of health care expenditure is general to most health systems. However, a system of expenditure control does not guarantee that resources are used efficiently. Expenditure limits merely act as a financial control system exercised on the total amount of resources available to the health sector. It does not ensure local accountability in terms of the efficient use of resources at the various tiers of control. As such, performance indicators were introduced to aid the monitoring of regional and district performance – which is, of course, a necessary first step towards implementing accountability procedures. They do, for example, allow the identification of outliers who might warrant further detailed analysis of their particular output.

Yet, while it is straightforward enough to monitor expenditure flows and even to tie these into measures of performance at an aggregate level concentrating on throughput, it is less simple to implement accountability procedures. This, after all, strikes at the heart of the self-regulatory role enjoyed by the medical profession. Therefore, it is perhaps not surprising that the UK performance indicators do in fact operate at a fairly aggregate level. All the present performance indicators are biased towards the monitoring of resources used by the NHS, as opposed to the monitoring of final outcomes – there is one exception, in that neonatal death rates are included in the current performance indicators package. In other words, the performance indicators introduced in the UK to monitor behaviour concentrate on expenditure levels and not on activity. But, of course, this does put the horse before the cart – if the NHS is to respond to local needs, then activity should dictate expenditure and not vice versa. Of course, this in itself raises problems in as much as need and activity have to be assessed. This is no easy matter, as earlier chapters have pointed out.

Not that the Department of Health and Social Security does not recognise the limitations of performance indicators. Indeed, they emphasise that no single indicator should be used to present 'good', 'bad' or 'efficient' and 'inefficient' behaviour. It is presumed that the indicators will do little more than point to pressing questions about unusual or atypical behaviour which will need further investigation (Department of Health and Social Security, 1983). In this respect, it is worth stating that aspects concerned with the health status of the region's population, the quality of care provided and the needs of the local population, although not covered by these indicators, remain fundamental to the assessment of performance in any hospital, district or region. Moreover, given the nature of the health care production process outlined above, it is not surprising that performance indicators will throw up variations in behaviour. Judgement is still required to assess what extent of variation is considered justified.

Given that, in principle, such measures are to be commended as a step in the right direction, it is worth while assessing their practical usefulness. In an attempt to do so, we shall take a closer look at the performance indicators introduced by the Department of Health and Social Security (DHSS) in 1983. These were presented in the publication *Performance Indicators: National Summary for 1981*. As published, they were crudely aggregated into five groups: clinical, financial, manpower, ambulance and estate management indicators. It is argued that these indicators are best presented as a complete package, for two reasons. First, the interrelationships that exist between the various indicators mean that a broad understanding of the use of resources in the various regions and districts will only be gained through analysis of the complete package. Second, as the indicators are drawn from various sources, a consistent picture can only be gained from a complete package.

Therefore, in judging how useful this set of performance indicators is, we must take account of its objective, which is to present a package of indicators which will aid individual regions and districts in the assessment of 'the efficiency of the services for which they are responsible' with regard to national comparisons.

In attempting to evaluate the performance indicators, we shall concentrate on the clinical, financial and manpower ones, partly as we judge these to be the most important and partly as these relate more directly to effectiveness issues. The indicators are each presented in separate sections. However, it is suggested that they are used not in isolation but in conjunction with the other sets of indicators. Consequently, we shall attempt to assess how reconcilable different sets of indicators are.

Let us first have a brief look at the clinical activity performance indicators. The first thing to note is that they are predominantly based on aggregate throughput measures – i.e. they tell us little about clinical effectiveness. They are concerned with measures such as length of stay, gross admission rate, waiting list per 1000 population, etc. The specialties are very broad – general medicine, general surgery, obstetrics, trauma and orthopaedics, and gynaecology – giving a high level of aggregation. In general, ten performance indicators are given for each specialty, although for general medicine and obstetrics only eight are presented – the missing indicators referring to waiting list information. In fact, the level of aggregation is high in another sense, inasmuch as it is intermediate rather than final outcome (measures of patient days rather than health status). Little attention is paid to severity and case-mix. It would be more helpful if such throughput measures were also analysed with regard to diagnostic categories and individual consultants' patient-mix.

Perhaps not surprisingly, given our earlier discussion on the nature of the health care production process, the performance indicators which remain in use in the UK appear to reflect a wide dimension of intermediate output in the sector. Given the specific lack of priority attached to any individual indicator, the failure to relate these aggregate indicators to diagnostic related groups (indeed, case-mix is only accounted for at an extremely crude level via the specialty definitions), the lack of consideration that case severity plays and the generally complex nature of intermediate production in this sector, it remains unclear as to what interpretation should be placed on these indicators. While throughput appears in a relatively large number of significant correlations, this is hardly surprising, since it is inextricably linked with both length of stay and turnover interval – i.e. two other performance measures.

The situation is superficially different when we turn to assess finances, because we compare everything in a common medium – cost. Given the greater emphasis implicitly being placed on value for money in the health care sector in recent years, one might expect the clinical performance indicators to be reconcilable with the financial indicators. However, currently in the UK system the clinical activity data are specialty-based while the financial data are hospital-based. At present, the cost of a service can not be related directly to activity rates.

The financial set of data are hospital-based, with a number of hospital categories being identified – acute, maternity and long-stay. Indeed, the acute hospitals were further subdivided into three groups: category A including wholly acute hospitals with more than 1000 beds along with partly acute hospitals larger than 200 beds; category B, which were acute hospitals with fewer than 50 beds; and category C, which were all other acute hospitals. We shall concentrate on category A.

The category A hospitals are ranked in terms of performance according to cost per case – not on the basis of actual cost per case, however, but rather on the basis of expected cost per case. The expected cost per case was obtained from a regression model of hospital costs which estimated costs for each specialty on the basis of an analysis of treatment and 'hotel' costs associated with the various specialties. No reference is made to the actual model used, although the results from the model are reported in the DHSS publication. To highlight the importance of underlying assumptions in considering performance indicators, we shall consider this model in a little more detail.

This is not the place to go into a detailed account of hospital cost modelling, but it should be pointed out that a number of problems remain to be resolved in this area. Cost functions are defined with regard to some concept of output. The DHSS model is based on the notion of bed-days as an output measure and therefore takes no account of, for example, differences in the quality of treatment or the effectiveness of treatment. In fact, there is no generally agreed definition of hospital output. Hospital costs must also be related to the particular production process associated with any hospital. Additionally, there are statistical problems (multicollinearity and heteroscedasticity) in the DHSS model, which make the results unreliable. Because no discussion of the model is presented with the performance indicators, the manager can not judge the usefulness of comparison based on expected length of stay figures. Summary information on performance is not useful if neither the objectives nor the assumptions are outlined.

Considering the fact that staff costs account for around 75% of the NHS revenue resources, it is a pity that the manpower performance indicators are not more useful. They are not at all compatible with the clinical activity or financial indicators. This is because the clinical data are specialty-specific, the financial data are hospital-specific and the manpower data are district-specific.

If it is found that a particular hospital is more expensive than other comparable hospitals, it would be helpful if the other indicators gave some idea whether this was due to its providing a 'better' nursing service or 'better' clinical service. The manpower statistics give a range of total and percentage breakdowns of staff categories, but more usefully include various ratios between nursing staff and cases, other staff and inpatient days. This is the closest that the indicators get to producing productivity ratios. Productivity ratios can be briefly defined as the ratio of a measure of output to a measure of one or more inputs. The simplest and most widely used form of productivity measurement relates output directly to input – e.g. the total number of employees. If this measure is used, the implication is that the objective is to maximise output per person, but without consideration of the associated total resource cost. Thus, this particular measure may differ across the sector, because each employee works different hours in different hospitals, or because different hospitals use different mixes of skilled and unskilled labour or different mixes of capital and labour. This is why it becomes important to reconcile financial and manpower data.

Of course, the major reconciliation has to be between inputs and outputs – i.e. manpower and clinical data. Notice here that the implicit output used in the performance indicators relates to patient-days. *Faute de mieux*, this is an intermediate or value-added measure: it does not relate to financial outcome – health status. Indeed, it is itself open to manipulation, as the number of days associated with a particular hospital visit will depend on over-all occupancy rates (i.e. capacity constraints), over-all case-mix and the severity of illness. In other words, it will be discretionary to some extent, the degree of discretion being a function of the medical condition involved. This will be largely a reflection of the difficulties in measuring output, although the difficulties in measuring inputs should not be ignored either.

It is worth noting at this point that one of the few analyses of a specific relationship between manpower and clinical data has highlighted that it is possible to determine the impact that staffing levels may have on health status. Mugford *et al.* (1988a) found that, after adjusting for differences in very-low-weight births, paediatric staffing ratios were inversely related to 'in-house' mortality rates. Further analysis showed that an inverse relationship between paediatric staffing and neonatal mortality was statistically significant before the introduction of a change in referral policy but not after (Mugford *et al.*, 1988b). Such studies clearly indicate the advantages of reconciling the information collected on inputs with that collected on outputs.

However, in general, the UK performance indicators are difficult to reconcile internally. It must be asked whether this is a problem peculiar to these specific performance indicators or whether there is some more fundamental difficulty. In particular, there may be problems even in attempting to consider the translation of cash into volumes of resources, let alone following through to final outcomes. It should be pointed out that we have deliberately concentrated on the medical and manpower indicators. There are also indicators dealing with the hotel aspects of health care. The comparative analysis of the costs of providing such services as catering and laundry to patients is obviously a much simpler task. However, it remains true that until we have better definitions and measures of health outcomes, a clearer idea of the relationship between utilisation rates and these outcomes, and a means to relate individual medical decision making to its associated economic consequences, it will remain difficult to analyse the fundamental activity of using resources to alter individual's health status.

CONCLUSIONS ON RECONCILIATION

It would appear, then, that the various indicators are not very reconcilable. This may be explained by the fact that the performance indicators are dictated by the financial considerations underlying the funding of the health care system rather than the efficiency with which final output is produced *per se*. It is because concern centres on funding and financing problems that emphasis is given to the use of existing data rather than placed on clearly outlining the objectives to be pursued and the collection of appropriate data to monitor explicitly the efficiency with which inputs are transformed into outputs. This leads to a focus on a fairly high level of aggregation: rather than focusing on activity levels and their relationship to health status, attention is focused on overall costs. Again, this relates to the fact that it is easier to regulate the costs of providing a health care system than to regulate the product – and, of course, here the product is activity levels rather than final outcome. As we noted above, this partly explains why the medical profession has obtained rights to self-regulation.

So let us conclude by quickly recapitulating and offering some observations. Health care and health care insurance cannot be provided efficiently in a market. Regulation is required with both commodities to overcome these market failures. Regulation leads to the monitoring of performance to ensure efficiency in production. The performance indicators recently introduced in the UK are an important recognition of the fact that regulation requires specific information. They are important in the sense that they foster a climate of comparison and inspection. It is against this background that their practical limitations should be assessed.

In discussions to date of health care systems and organisations generally, there has not been enough recognition given to the fact that there are two commodities produced in the health care sector – health care and health care insurance. Regulation and therefore performance monitoring have concentrated on the costs of providing health care insurance rather than health care *per se*. With health care insurance, regulation has taken the form of government's (or third party's) underwriting the cost of provision of health care. At present we are witnessing increasing monitoring and control of these costs. With health care itself, regulation has taken the form of professional self-regulation. By its very nature such regulation makes external (i.e. governmental) control and monitoring problematical. However, if the form and character of such self-regulation does not respond to changing environmental conditions (such as the increasing regulation and monitoring of the costs of health care insurance), it will become increasingly threatened by alternative forms of regulations (e.g. litigation). The choice seems largely between changing the existing character of self-regulation to encompass more explicit forms of control and monitoring (e.g. peer group review of medical performance) or that the self-regulation of medical conduct will become undermined by the domination of the regulation of the economic aspects associated with the provision of health care. Fundamental to this choice is the point that, because of the acceptance that markets fail, the rights to self-regulation held by the medical profession are essentially to protect the patient; they are not there to protect the monopoly position of the medical profession. The closing of professional ranks (e.g. over the release of information) or any tendency towards defensive practices does not aid the agency relationship (which is founded on trust between the doctor and the patient) and will, in the long run, not help to secure the self-regulatory role of the profession. Such regulation has to be self-supporting if overall efficiency is to be gained in the health care sector, given the inter-relationships that exist between health care and health care insurance.

The difficulty is that performance, at least with respect to health care *per se*, is being monitored at the wrong level (i.e. it is the aggregate costs associated with health care insurance with which concern lies). This will inevitably lead to distortions in provision and dissatisfaction over the provision. Finances can not determine the form of health care except in a very crude manner – needs remain to be defined. Given the medical profession's monopoly over information, it is inevitable that they will be intricately involved in defining needs. If they do not do so sensibly, then they risk losing their rights to self-regulation. If current trends continue, there are strong incentives to standardise treatment patterns – possibly even at the lower end of provision – and thereby reduce medical practice variations, *irrespective* of whether such reduction improves efficiency or not. Monitoring the performance of health care costs has the accompanying problem that the impact on care is not necessarily on the side of improvement. Slimming down costs may have unforeseen impacts on both health and health care. For example, it is likely that the necessary capacity planned to meet the unforeseen aspects associated with the prognostic and diagnostic uncertainties that underlie the production process will be squeezed out of the system.

Yet all of this is an open question. At least, the monitoring of costs has introduced a climate in which comparison is emphasised. The medical profession have for far too long disregarded not only the practice of self-government, but also the nature of their rights to self-government. Clearly, more information is required on efficiacy and effectiveness. Even acknowledging the individualistic nature of the production process in this sector, not enough attention has been given to the definition of acceptable levels of medical practice variation. If the profession does not act, that acceptable level of variation may be defined outside the profession as being close to zero.

The medical profession has to recognise that its agency role underlies the rights to self-government. Given the assumption that it is activity that should dictate performance levels rather than costs, information should focus on clinical activity at the individualistic level. Analysis of variations in medical practice should be incorporated within the self-regulatory procedures of the medical profession. Indeed, this has to be the case if performance monitoring is to be reconciled with the actual production process. In this way regulation of health care costs should support and not lead the monitoring of performance in this sector. Variation in practice has to be accepted, but within limits. If it should prove necessary to choose between the doctors and the cost containers, it is better that the medical profession define these limits than have them imposed as a secondary consequence of monitoring the costs of provision. This is not to suggest that difficult choices will not have to be made. But surely it is better that such choices are made with the best possible information, with clear definitions and with the objective of providing effective *and* efficient health care.

ACKNOWLEDGEMENTS

I should like to thank Alastair Gray and the editors for helpful comments on this chapter. Also, thanks to Brian Ferguson for research assistance on some of the material contained herein. Liability remains with the author. I also wish to thank the Nuffield Provincial Hospitals' Trust for financial support.

REFERENCES

Arrow, K. (1963). Uncertainty and the welfare economics of medical care. *American Economic Review*, **53**, 941–73

Berki, S. (1983). The design of case-based hospital payment systems. *Medical Care*, **21**, 1–13

Department of Health and Social Security (1983). *Performance Indicators: National Summary for 1981*. DHSS, London

Evans, R. G. (1981). Incomplete vertical integration; the distinctive structure of the health care industry. In van der Gaag, J. and Perlman, M. (Eds.), *Health, Economics and Health Economics*. North-Holland, Amsterdam

Evans, R. G. (1984). *Strained Mercy: The Economics of the Canadian Health Care System*. Butterworths, Toronto

Hall, M. and Whinston, C. (1959). The ambiguous notion of efficiency. *Economic Journal*, **69**, 71–88

Harris, J. (1977). The internal organisation of the hospital; some economic implications. *The Bell Journal of Economics*, **8**, 467–82

HMSO (1979). *Royal Commission on the National Health Service*, cmnd. 7615. HMSO, London

McGuire, A., Henderson, J. and Mooney, G. (1988). *The Economics of Health Care: An Introductory Text*. Routledge and Kegan Paul, London

Mugford, M. *et al.* (1988a). Factors affecting the outcome of maternity care. I. The relationship between staffing and perinatal birth at the hospital of birth. *Journal of Epidemiology and Community Health*, **42**, 157–69

Mugford, M. *et al.* (1988b). Factors affecting the outcome of maternity care. II. Neonatal outcomes and resources beyond the hospital birth. *Journal of Epidemiology and Community Health*, **42**, 170–6

Weisbrod, B. (1978). Comment on M. Pauly. In Greenberg, W. (Ed.), *Competition in the Health Care Sector.* Proceedings of a conference sponsored by the Bureau of Economics, Federal Trade Commission. Aspen Systems, Germanstown

CHAPTER 7

The Dog in the Night-time: Medical Practice Variations and Health Policy

Robert G. Evans

INTRODUCTION

Knowing is not the same as doing. The most striking fact about the large and extensively documented variations in patterns of medical practice, throughout the developed world, is the minimal impact this information has had on health policy.

For many years, students of health care utilisation have been demonstrating that per capita rates of surgical procedures, hospital utilisation and medical service use vary widely across large and small geographic areas, and that servicing patterns for particular conditions vary among both institutions and individual practitioners. These differences, moreover, do not appear to be explicable in terms of the needs or characteristics of the populations served – or, at least, such explanations have not been found.

Similar observations emerge in every country studied, despite the substantial differences in their systems for organising, regulating and reimbursing health services. The research findings are really quite remarkable in their scale and consistency. Yet nowhere has there been any significant adaptation in regulation or reimbursement.

Earlier on in the development of this field of investigation, one might have assumed that the explanation was simple ignorance. Providers of and payers for services may merely have been unaware of the existence of such variations – after all, research is expected to reveal the unknown. Furthermore, particular findings require time for confirmation and general acceptance by the research community, and for dissemination among those whose decisions and behaviour might be expected to change.

But it is now *20 years* since the first studies in the English-speaking countries began to focus attention on this phenomenon (Pearson *et al.*, 1968; Lewis, 1969; Bunker, 1970; Vayda, 1973). And it would be wrong to assume that, even in the late 1960s agencies responsible for reimbursing health services had no idea as to the variety of servicing patterns for which they were paying (Note 1). The academic literature has grown substantially in range and sophistication, as has awareness of the consistency and pervasiveness of medical practice variations. But to argue that policy makers have been waiting, all this time, for the research literature to become sufficiently secure to support action is to suggest that those responsible are not merely sleeping but dead.

In this chapter we explore an alternative position. We assume that those responsible for health policy are in fact quite aware of medical practice variations, and have been, in general terms at least, for many years. But there are very good reasons why they have not reacted to the accumulating evidence. The belief that they *would* react, once provided with the relevant information, is based on underlying assumptions as to the objectives of health policy, and the instruments and constraints through which it is shaped, which may be inappropriate. The objectives of health policy are typically postulated, tacitly, through a relatively straightforward extension of the objectives of individuals, in their roles as citizens and actual or potential patients. This extension is certainly incomplete, and may be unsound (Note 2).

If this alternative view is correct, it has implications for the likely effect, or lack of it, from further research on medical practice variations. We close with some consideration of the pressures which *do* seem to be driving changes in health policies, and the prospects for better informing this process through the application of the substantial knowledge which has unquestionably been generated by such research.

THE OBJECTIVES OF HEALTH CARE

The dominant view of health care – and, by extension, of the health care system – remains an instrumental one. Patients seek care in order to be relieved of some actual or perceived, present or potential, 'dis-ease'. The care itself is not directly of value; it is generally inconvenient, often painful or frightening. As a thought experiment, one could ask a representative patient (or oneself) whether he/she would prefer to have or contemplate a condition perceived as requiring care, plus the best conceivable care for that condition, completely free of all direct or indirect costs, or would prefer simply not to have the condition. The answer is in most cases obvious. Care is not a 'good' in the usual sense, but a 'bad' or 'regrettable', made 'necessary' by the even more regrettable circumstances of 'dis-ease' (Note 3).

It follows that patients want to receive *effective* health care, i.e. care which they 'need' in the sense that there is a reasonable expectation that such care will have a positive impact on their health (Note 4). Ineffective, unnecessary care is of no, or negative, value to the patient, as well as a complete waste of the resources required to produce it. But the judgement of effectiveness requires patients to have access to 'technical' information, about the relationship between their conditions and the potential effects of a multitude of different intervention manoeuvres – commodities and services, in different doses or combinations.

The expansion of medical and biological knowledge, over the last century at least, has led most societies to judge this access impossible, for the unaided 'consumer'. The regulatory structure of the 'professions' creates special privileges and obligations for various classes of personnel providing health care, in the expectation that they will make appropriate decisions on the patient's behalf. Even when organised as self-employed entrepreneurs, earning profits from fees for their services, they are expected to be motivated by the patient's interest, to run 'not-only-for-profit' businesses (Evans, 1984, Ch. 7). Similarly, the institutions providing care, such as hospitals, are typically organised on a not-for-profit basis, so that the interests of owners in profits shall not threaten the interests of patients who are not in a position to defend themselves (Note 5).

The special social and legal status of the 'professional', as agent for the patient, has a very long history in Europe and North America, and is deeply entrenched in statute and custom. During the twentieth century, these societies have intervened in a second way to protect the individual patient against the increasing financial burdens of health care. The reimbursement of providers of care is now in developed countries almost entirely carried out collectively, either directly by governments or through various forms of 'social' or private insurance funds. All such, however, are highly regulated by the state, even in the rhetorically 'free enterprise' USA.

Implicit in both the professionalised provision of health care and its collective payment is the initial assumption of instrumentality. The professional provider is granted extraordinary privileges and undertakes special obligations, in order that he/she can provide, not simply the care the patient is willing and able to pay for, but also the care he/she believes the patient needs. The professional provider does not simply meet a market demand in the most profitable manner possible – that is the role of the quack. If the care is inappropriate to the patient's condition, the professional should not be providing it, whether or not the patient is willing to pay (Note 6).

Payers, whether public or private, are implicitly or explicitly obligated to reimburse only 'needed' care. The provider's judgement of need is generally accepted in individual cases, but payers in different countries

have imposed a variety of regulatory and budgetary constraints intended to limit the volume of care provided and paid for. In an earlier
day, the complex apparatus of 'deterrent' charges imposed on patients,
which still characterises the insurance scene in the USA, was believed to
have the potential to discourage selectively the 'unnecessary' use of
care, although it is now more generally recognised as embodying
primarily wealth redistributional objectives.

The restriction of reimbursement to the services of particular classes
of providers is a reflection of an assumption that some types of services
(e.g. those of cardiac surgeons) are inherently more 'needed' than others
(e.g. those of massage practitioners) – or at least less likely to be
provided when not 'needed'. The consequences of error, in (non-)
provision or in (non-)reimbursement, are also rather different.

This rather simplistic characterisation of the intent of the health care
system yields one of the most basic objectives of health policy – to
provide and pay for needed services. There is, of course, a lot more
besides (Note 7), but providers and payers alike would generally agree,
as would the general public in their various roles as voters, taxpayers
and potential or actual patients. Moreover, the basic institutional structure of health care provision and finance, in all developed nations, only
makes logical sense on the basis of some such objective.

THE EMBARRASSMENT OF VARIATIONS IN PATTERNS OF CARE

Given this objective, the implications of variations in practice patterns
are obvious. Either some regions, institutions, practitioners are doing
things they should not be doing, or others are leaving undone things
they should be doing. In either case, some change is called for. *Laissez
faire*, by both the professional community and the reimbursement
agencies, is leading either to unnecessary servicing, with associated
risks to patients as well as waste of human and financial resources, or to
underservicing and the failure to meet legitimate needs. One way or
another, the observation of systematic and persistent variations is *prima
facie* evidence of a system of care which is not meeting its objectives.

Other explanations, of course, have been offered. It is possible that
practice variations reflect genuine differences in the 'needs' of different
populations, resulting from differences in environment, life-style, genetic endowment – all the various factors which can be shown or
hypothesised to affect human health. Less defensibly, but understand-
ably, they may reflect cultural differences in expectations or beliefs
about health and health care – although these are at least interactive
with the patterns of health care delivery themselves. Providers are more

likely to offer what their patients expect and believe in, but patients learn to expect and believe in what their providers offer.

The progress of research has steadily stripped away the various *ad hoc* rationalisations. No one study has been conclusive, and in any case analysis of non-experimental data can never eliminate the possibility of effects from unmeasured confounding variables (Note 8). But the accumulation of evidence has now reached the point at which most observers would regard the justification of variations by 'different needs' as an essentially circular argument (Note 9).

The point to notice, however, is that the observed pattern of response by the clinical community is inconsistent with the basic postulate of policy objectives. If providers of care were really concerned solely to offer their patients the most effective care possible, they would have seized upon even the earliest evidence of variations as grounds for concern and for further study – by themselves. Instead, the physicians, in particular, who have been engaged in this field of research have spent 20 years trying to attract the attention of their colleagues in clinical practice, and to penetrate the screen of ignorance, indifference, and rationalisation which has greeted their findings (Note 10).

But the response by those responsible for reimbursement and administration is even more puzzling. Policy makers at this level are thoroughly familiar with the type of statistical evidence from which medical practice variations emerge, and furthermore have been under strong pressure for most of the last two decades (depending on the country) to rationalise the provision of health care, make it more efficient and, most specifically, hold down its costs. If their objectives were really to oversee and reimburse the delivery of effective health care, and to contain costs by identifying and weeding out the ineffective, they should not only be responding to the accumulating evidence, but also be among its most enthusiastic sponsors. They have not, and are not.

The question, then, is: what *are* these respective policy-making groups trying to achieve or maintain, or at least what objectives would be consistent with their behaviour? If effectiveness of care is not the only, or even the dominant, goal, what are the competitors? To oversimplify a broad and complex set of ideas, we focus on two additional summary or short-hand objectives – cost control and autonomy.

AFTER PUBLICATION, WHAT NEXT?

Consider the logical sequence from (awareness of) research findings to policy decisions. Once one moves beyond the stage of defensive rationalisation, several kinds of questions arise.

First and most obviously, if variations represent evidence of inappropriate care, *which* care is inappropriate? Are the regions, or institutions, or practitioners with high rates over-providing, or are the low ones under-providing, or does the 'best' rate lie somewhere in the middle? (or beyond either end?)

Second, if the direction of the appropriate adjustment can be determined, who is responsible for taking action? Health policy, as noted above, may be made by regulators, by payers, by providers collectively through the self-regulatory process, through hospital staffs, or through the professional literature, or by individual clinicians in deciding what to do in particular circumstances.

And finally, though clearly connected with the second point, what forms of actions are appropriate? Professional guidelines? limitations on payment? practice review? publicity in professional journals? in the press? . . . , and so on.

This range of questions was clearly addressed, explicitly or implicitly, from the beginning of research on practice variations. With understandable diffidence, however, researchers in commenting on their own and others' findings emphasised the first question – the impossibility of inferring, from the observation of variations alone, the relationship between what is and what ought to be. In the absence of such additional information, of course, one cannot determine what policy changes should occur. The inference drawn was that, in fact, nothing should be done – further research was necessary.

Further research has, of course, been done; the study of medical practice variations has become almost a subdiscipline of health services research (Copenhagen Collaborating Center, 1987; Paul-Shaheen *et al.*, 1987; Ham, 1988). But by 1986 Chassin *et al.* were still making the same point – as does Wennberg (1988). One cannot tell whether the high regions are too high, or the low regions are too low, so any policy intervention is premature. 'More research' has greatly improved the documentation of the basic phenomenon, and has eliminated a number of hypothetical explanations, but has brought researchers no nearer to any useful conclusion on the basic policy issue – what is to be done?

And yet the study of medical practice variations has never been carried out simply for the inherent fascination of collecting and tabulating numbers, '. . . a spectator sport for epidemiologists' (Jennett, 1988, p. 31). Its practitioners have always believed that they were engaged in a substantial exercise to improve the quality of medical care, by changing patterns of practice and linking them more closely to the underlying needs of the population served. Why, then, is so little progress made on this most basic point?

In part, of course, the answer is that the task of defining the 'needs' of whole populations is inherently very difficult. Again, more, bigger and better research is needed. But it is also evident that the 'too much/too little' axis is the intersection between clinical and economic motives. It is here that the objectives of payers and providers are most explicitly in conflict. If unusually high servicing rates represent 'excess', and if they can be pushed down, then the costs of health care will fall, or at least escalate less rapidly. Unfortunately, and by elementary arithmetic, so will the incomes of providers. Conversely, 'underservicing' implies that more should be done – and paid for.

PRACTICE PATTERNS ARE ALSO PAYMENT PATTERNS – AND INCOME PATTERNS

This conflict of interest is fundamental, and unavoidable, so long as providers are reimbursed, through whatever channels, for doing things and not for not doing them. Providers and payers may declare a common interest in ensuring the availability of effective care for the populations they serve. Who can be against 'quality' and 'access'? But their interests with respect to costs are diametrically opposed. What one pays, the other earns.

Thus, we find a distinct split emerging in the commentary on practice variations. On one side are those concerned with the payers' problem, who emphasise the linkage between 'utilisation review' (UR) and cost control. Go and find out what clinicians are doing, and make them stop. Then we will not have to pay so much, either to them or to those whose activities they direct or set in motion. Webber and Goldbeck (1984), in a collection of American essays on the potential for cost control by private reimbursers, put the point clearly:

> 'While there is no intimation that all physicians should practice in a like manner, there is no medical excuse for the variation in practice patterns that now exists, and UR can be expected to narrow of [sic] the accepted range of variations.... The development of outcome-validated standards will be the next great advance toward a more uniformly high-quality, less wasteful, delivery system' [p. 89].

It is taken for granted that the current delivery system, at least in the USA, *is* wasteful, and that variations in practice patterns are one form of evidence – though by no means the only one. McClure and Shaller (1984) draw the same inference:

> '... differences in provider efficiency may account for much and perhaps

the majority of the observed variations in per capita expenditure rates. . . . To the extent that wide variations in provider efficiency are substantiated by further research, it should be possible to constrain costs by improving efficiency . . .' [p. 127].

Nor is the assumption restricted to the USA, a clear outlier with respect to health care costs (Scheiber and Poullier, 1988). The *Economist* for 17 December 1988, in an article headed 'Fallible Doctors, Patient's Dilemma', draws heavily on the practice variations literature, and concludes that: 'More information about competing treatments promises to improve healthcare and also to slow the rapid rise in health costs.'

Enthoven has, in fact, addressed this issue on both sides of the Atlantic (1985, 1988a, b). His concern has been to promote structural reorganisations of health care delivery systems which will create both opportunities and incentives for reimbursers to collect and use more information on, *inter alia*, patterns of medical care utilisation. His argument for reorganisation shares some common ground with a central theme of this chapter, that the motivations and/or authority of those who now administer and pay for health care do not encourage them to promote the provision of effective and efficient health care. In particular, there is no overriding reason for them to react to the evidence on variations – in the US, the UK or anywhere else.

The initial question, however, as to whether high rates represent overuse or low rates represent underuse, has not, in fact, been answered explicitly, except in a very limited number of cases. Webber and Goldbeck (1984) refer to outcome-validated studies as in the future, and for the most part they still are. What has happened is that there has been a shift in the burden of proof. With increasing suspicion about the net payoff to health care in general, at least at the margin – the famous 'flat-of-the-curve' medicine – the feeling has grown (among non-providers) that 'when in doubt, don't' is a more appropriate decision rule than 'when in doubt, do'. The continued rapid growth of costs in the USA, and the steadily escalating pressure from the health care sector in other countries where cost control has been more successful, have encouraged this shift in attitude.

But the health care researchers, many of them physicians, who have been the primary contributors to the variations literature, appear to have ambiguous feelings towards cost control. Wennberg, whose name is virtually synonymous with the field, is willing to accept limitation of costs *in hospitals* as a legitimate objective (Wennberg, 1984), but states: 'The shift of . . . patients to the ambulatory setting will neither disrupt the patient–physician relationship nor have a significant negative economic impact on physicians' [p. 26].

Yet the question of whether particular procedures should be performed on an inpatient or an ambulatory basis is a minute and relatively trivial part of the variations literature. The central question has always been whether the procedures should be performed at all – a question which does directly affect the income of the physician.

More recently, Gabel *et al.* (1988) have noted the implications of the very rapid rise of costs in the ambulatory care sector in the USA. They show that the reduction in inpatient utilisation has simply transferred costs from one sector to another, and has had no effect at all on the overall rate of escalation. The lower-income employees of hospitals – housekeepers, dietary workers, practical nurses and attendants – may have lost ground; but the upper echelons of the health care industry have seen an expansion, not a shrinkage, in their income opportunities.

While Wennberg appears ambiguous about cost control, others are more forthright. Chassin *et al.* (1986, p. 289) express their concern that, if physicians do not respond to the growing evidence, others with different motives will do so: 'Policy makers seem ready to equate high use with inappropriate use. Such an assumption is ill-informed and dangerous.' They urge their colleagues to take control of the issue, to keep it out of the hands of the cost-cutters. Jennett (1988) likewise urges surgeons to collect more data themselves on the patterns and outcomes of their activities, rather than 'responding defensively to inadequate data from others' (p. 30). Perhaps the most blunt of all is Bowen (1987, p. 1580): 'Studies of practice style should have but one purpose, to help doctors become better doctors.' If the American Secretary for Health and Human Services saw any scope for containing his Department's budget, he certainly did not admit it.

Jennett emphasises that surgeons are unlikely to take notice of data other than those collected and interpreted by themselves or other credible clinicians – particularly other surgeons. Buck (1988) goes further, and states that the 'enthusiasm and trust of consultants' is a precondition for the very *performance* of peer audit studies, let alone for their information to have any impact on clinical practice.

If these views are correct, they point up a central dilemma for the use of variations data in cost control. It may be that one *cannot* use detailed data on practice patterns simultaneously to improve the quality of care and to reduce costs. It is naïve to imagine that cost reduction can ever be anything but confrontational; the only difference among health care systems is the degree of centralisation or decentralisation of that confrontation (Evans *et al.*, 1989b). Thus, if variations research becomes an input to the cost control process, it will automatically lose the 'enthusiasm and trust' of clinicians, and be greeted instead with even more intense hostility and suspicion (Note 11). The only way out of this dilemma may be that chosen by Wennberg, to try to enlist the co-operation of physicians in eliminating other health workers' jobs (Note 12).

Wennberg's own proposals for action (1984) emphasise the central role of physicians, both individually and collectively, in defining and managing the appropriate response. The corporate reimbursers of care, who in the scenarios of Enthoven, or Webber and Goldbeck, were to be the driving forces reshaping medical practice, are reduced to supplying their data to central agencies under physician control.

This emphasis could reflect a pragmatic judgement that only physician-led and -controlled institutions have any real prospect of changing the way in which physicians practise medicine. But the general tone of Wennberg's work seems to support a stronger conclusion – that, in fact, his primary interest is in improving the quality and effectiveness of medical practice, and that he has less concern for cost control *per se*.

The policy implication drawn by most researchers on practice variations is that resources should be *redeployed* within the health care sector so as to respond to actual patterns of patient need. Shrinkage, or slower growth, of the health care sector is *not* recommended. Implicitly, this assumes that, to the extent that variations identify situations of over-servicing, there are, must be, under-serviced people and problems somewhere else. The priorities for use of freed-up resources within the health care system are greater than any conceivable, or at least likely, use they might have outside health care. This assumption has generally seemed self-evident to those trained in, and earning their livings from, any branch of health care.

Furthermore, most researchers in this field seem to feel that the process of response to the variations evidence should be thoroughly under the control of clinicians and the organisations representing them, which would seem to guarantee that the overall incomes/costs of providers will not be adversely affected. Cost control is a central part of health care policy for payers and providers alike. Both want to control costs. But one group wants to hold them down, the other to push them up – independently of the question of the effectiveness of particular procedures (Evans, 1988b). To the extent that providers retain control of policies responding to practice variations, *The Economist* will be dis-appointed.

Well, so what? Why should it be of any great significance to explore the personal views and preferences of particular investigators? Surely their work speaks for itself? From the point of view of payers for health care, formulating reimbursement policy, it does not. The opinions and values of the generators of research become extremely important in its interpretation, and thus form a significant part of the political environ-ment constraining policy makers. For the moment, however, we shall defer the discussion of this point, because it interacts with the second major policy objective, physician autonomy.

CLINICAL FREEDOM AS MEANS OR AS END

The intense dedication of physicians to their professional independence, both individual and collective, has few parallels in the modern world. As work environments have made people increasingly interdependent, even in medicine, physicians have nevertheless managed to retain an extraordinary degree of autonomy in the management of their own work, and in their entitlement to call upon a vast array of other social resources as they see fit. In principle, they admit accountability only to their peers for their actions; in practice, even that form of control is rarely in evidence.

The demise of clinical freedom and the 'proletarianisation' of physicians has frequently been predicted. It would seem to follow logically, from the increasing interdependence of the different components of the health care system, and the greater co-ordination required for the care of patients in a world of ever more complex technology. Yet the profession has managed to maintain its essentially autonomous status, and to stave off threats from a number of quarters.

At one time 'socialised medicine' was perceived as the great enemy; physicians were all to be converted into *de facto* civil servants. The various experiences of the UK, Canada, and Sweden have made it clear that, at least up until the present, reimbursement of care in large part or in total from public funds is quite compatible with maintenance of clinical autonomy. (Economic autonomy, however, is another matter.)

The current threat is from the private sector. Within the last decade, physicians in the USA have been 'blind-sided by capitalism', and the challenge of the marketplace is still being fought out in that country (Starr, 1982; Bock, 1988; Scovern, 1988). But the American experience is unique, and the steam seems to be going out of the current round of 'competitive' policies there (Weiner *et al.*, 1987; Ginzburg, 1988) (Note 13).

A more fundamental challenge may yet be mounted from the technological side. With the progress of artificial intelligence, much of the physician's role could become obsolete (Rennels and Shortliffe, 1987). Here too, however, control over the social and economic context of practice, maintained through the regulatory system, will probably permit physicians to keep control of the new technology, and use it to complement, not to substitute for, their skills. The successful suppression of the nurse practitioner, a technologically superior substitute for the physician in a number of roles, is illustrative (Record, 1981; Spitzer, 1984; Lomas and Barer, 1986).

This latter example demonstrates one instrumental role of legally protected autonomy; it has served powerfully to defend the profession (and other professions) against external threats to their economic position. Physicians appear to be selected and socialised to value autonomy very highly for its own sake (Shapiro, 1978), but it serves other collective purposes as well.

However, the usual justification offered to the rest of society, as to why this degree of autonomy should be tolerated and institutionally protected, is also instrumental. The patient will receive better care. The (properly trained) physician who is completely free to exercise his/her own expert judgement, in interpreting the circumstances and recommending/providing interventions, will, in general, achieve better outcomes. The uniqueness of individuals, the complexity of their problems, do not permit any feasible 'cookbook' or predetermined responses.

Mistakes will, of course, be made, because no one is perfect, not even the highly trained clinician. And even the best of care sometimes yields bad results; powerful interventions have powerful side-effects. Or the patient's circumstances may be such that even the best possible care cannot remedy them. But, in general, on balance, the best results will follow from ensuring that the clinician is highly trained and has access to whatever support staff and equipment he/she may demand, and then letting him/her alone to get on with the job.

It is important to be clear, however, that this is an *instrumental* argument. It accepts implicitly that autonomy, clinical freedom, is a privilege granted to physicians (and, to a lesser extent, other professionals) by the rest of the community, who tolerate the suspension of normal processes of accountability. They do so because (to the extent that they think about it at all) they accept the proposition that this freedom results, on balance, in patients receiving more appropriate care than they would under conceivable alternatives. (Most people have more confidence in physicians than in administrators and bureaucrats.)

The observation of widespread and large variations in clinical practice strikes at the heart of this argument. Physicians, and health care providers more generally, claim that they draw on an extensive base of both scientifically grounded knowledge and accumulated art and skill in selecting the interventions they will recommend and undertake. If their actual performance is, in fact, all over the map, if different practitioners respond to essentially similar (or indeed actually similar: Renaud *et al.*, 1980) circumstances in very different ways, it is hard to believe that each is right in his own way. The presumption that diagnosis and therapy have a scientific basis, which providers know (and act upon) and others do not, cannot be reconciled with patterns of provision which appear arbitrary and capricious.

The blow is not in itself fatal. One could still argue that, even if clinical freedom, absence of accountability, results in patterns of practice which are wildly at variance with patient needs, it may still yield results which are better than any known alternative. But this is an eminently contestable proposition. *Some* form of systematisation of practice seems an obvious alternative. If clinicians really support clinical freedom, defend it to the death, only because of their commitment to the well-being of their patients, then they would presumably respond to the variations evidence with deep concern. They might not abandon their commitment to autonomy, but would at least call it into question, and make a serious effort to find out whether some form of evaluation and co-ordination of their activities might yield better results.

In fact, they have not done so. Reactions have been defensive, or dismissive. Jennett (1988, p. 30) refers to one commentator who actually *welcomed* the evidence of practice variations as indicative of the survival of clinical freedom in the NHS! The obvious implication is that autonomy is valued for its own sake, independently of its contribution to patient outcomes. As *The Economist* (1988) pointed out: 'In attempting to draw up any sort of medical guidelines, governments face opposition from the medical profession. Doctors call it "cookbook medicine"'.

But if providers, and particularly physicians, attach such great importance to autonomy for its own sake, *even if the exercise of autonomy leads to patterns of practice which are, on the face of it at least, wasteful or harmful to patients*, this has important implications for the role of evidence in health policy. To the practitioner, variations in practice patterns are simply not a problem. Jennett's unnamed commentator was being quite honest, and may have been speaking for the majority of his colleagues. The preservation of autonomy is more important than the mitigation of its possible adverse consequences for patients; and no amount of additional evidence will reduce opposition to 'cookbook medicine' (Note 14).

This possibility finds indirect support in the arguments being made to their colleagues by students of medical practice variations in the USA. Brook *et al.* (1984) are quite explicit in pointing to the threats from payers and regulators.

> 'Times, however, are changing . . . the unchallenged position of organized medicine in choosing the future direction of the health care system is eroding. If the profession is to have a strong voice in the future, it must set about to examine within a clinical framework its past and present acts as a means of drawing lessons for the future' [p. 71].

The same note is struck in Chassin *et al.* (1986). 'The unchallenged position of organized medicine in choosing the future of the health care system', of course, disappeared a long time ago outside the USA, and, even there, the mid-1960s witnessed the arrival of some new players on the scene. But the point is clear. If physicians do not take collective action to rationalise their own behaviour, others will seize on this evidence and use it for their own ends.

Those ends will certainly include limitation on health expenditures, bad in itself for providers, and will be sought through some form of external control on practice independence, also *per se* offensive. Nor are they likely to give due weight to the complexities of maintaining the 'quality of patient care', in defence of which, of course, physicians struggle to protect and enhance both their freedom from external accountability and their share of national resources. It is precisely because the observation of practice variations, and of physicians' non-response to them, undermines the credibility of this latter claim, that some response is called for.

DISAGREEMENT IS NOT UNCERTAINTY

But the problem faced by clinicians, in coming to terms with the implications of diversity, has unfortunately been somewhat obscured by the context within which it has been placed, and even the choice of language used to describe it. The collectivity of clinicians, and of clinical knowledge, has been confused, rhetorically, with the individual. The label of 'clinical uncertainty' may be misleading in this regard.

The evidence that variations in practice patterns are most pronounced among particular procedures, for which there is least agreement on the indications for performance or on effectiveness, is consistent with the interpretation that the profession as a whole has no coherent view as to what should be done in these circumstances. In a sense, the *group* is uncertain; if you ask its members, you get different answers.

But it does not follow that each, or even any, *individual clinician* is in the slightest degree uncertain. He/she may be, but the variations data do not show it. Deep and intense disagreement, on the basis of strongly held views, will also yield a diversity of behaviour.

Now of course, if medical practice has a fundamental scientific, or even more generally rational, basis, then presumably there exists a 'right' and a 'wrong' approach to each situation, although there may be a continuum of responses, with no very sharp dividing line, rather than a clear-cut 'either/or'. Current knowledge may not permit the identification of that 'correct' intervention, but presumably there is also a 'best' or a range of acceptable, interpretations of current evidence (Note 15). Collective uncertainty exists if that range of acceptable interpretations is diverse and/or not strongly held.

When Wennberg (1988, p. 32) says: 'Too often physicians do not know what works best for the health of their patients', he presupposes the existence of an approach that 'works best', which either is known or could be discovered by further research. When practices vary, some at least of those who 'do not know' are doing the wrong things. But the critical question is: Do the individual clinicians concerned *know* that they do not know? Or are they firmly convinced of the effectiveness of their current practices, even though their convictions have no basis in generally accepted scientific fact?

The language of 'uncertainty' suggests the former. But if that were so, individual clinicians would react with enthusiasm and gratitude to new information which promised to resolve their uncertainties. They would not celebrate the evidence of their diversity, and they would certainly not have to be threatened with worse alternatives, the bogeyman of lay control, in order to persuade them to take an interest. Most people do not like to remain uncertain about the effects of what they are doing, and responsible clinicians, convinced of the importance of their work to the lives and well-being of their patients, are surely no different.

However, the actual response suggests rather a clinical community which not only attaches a high value to its autonomy, but also whose members are in the main quite confident in their practice. The surgeons who scrawl their surgical signatures across Wennberg's data sets, the hospital-prone physicians identified by Roos *et al.* (1986) who maintain the hospital industry of rural Manitoba, are not at all uncertain about the rightness of what they are doing (Note 16).

If challenged to explain how everyone can be right, while being so different, they would probably dismiss the question. Statistics are notoriously unreliable, and, anyway, every patient is unique. Jennett's anonymous commentator, celebrating the diversity of practice, does not appear to have employed the more sophisticated argument that a diversity of behaviour in the face of genuine uncertainty may be an efficient search strategy for finding the best approach. Variations are a GOOD THING, either in themselves, or as evidence of clinical freedom, which is unquestionably a GOOD THING. There is no problem.

WHAT DO YOU MEAN, 'WE'?

Or at least there is no problem unless 'outsiders' – those responsible for paying the bills – create a problem. Brook *et al.* (1984) threaten that times are changing, as does the *Economist*. The former urge clinicians, in essence: curb your individual autonomy to protect your collective autonomy. Circle the wagons; the Indians are coming. Again, however, there is a confusion of individual and collective interest.

To academic physicians, for whom research and clinical progress are an important part of self-image and life-style, 'cookbook medicine' as such is not a threat. They and their colleagues will write the cookbooks. That in itself will be a major intellectual and methodological challenge; and if they do not like the results, or as new knowledge emerges, they will rewrite the book. They will still be 'the experts' – which is a good thing to be.

But the ordinary community practitioner will have little or no input to the process of defining practice standards. Whether those standards are based on randomised trials, consensus conferences, retrospective research or expert panels, only an élite minority of the profession will, or can, be involved.

That would not be so bad if the standards were, as in the past, just an expression of good intentions, having no practical effect on the behaviour of the average clincian. But the whole point of the 'circle the wagons' argument is that, finally, practice patterns really have to change. Physicians have to be serious about self-government, and to take some form of collective action against non-conforming members. At the very least, that requires monitoring their behaviour and bringing aberrant behaviour to the attention of the practitioners concerned. If this does not yield a response, further intervention would be necessary.

Furthermore, the scale of the variations in practice patterns identified in the literature implies that this would involve not merely harassing a handful of dubious actors, but also changing the behaviour of a significant proportion of the practitioner community. There is no precedent for an effort on this scale, let alone for its success.

From the point of view of the practitioner-in-the-street, the 'cure' offered by Brook *et al.* (1984) may not look much better than the disease. The sacrifice of autonomy is as great; the only difference is that it is sacrificed to members of his/her own profession, and not to 'bureaucrats' or 'laymen'. But the functional difference is very small. After all, as every clinician knows, physicians in administrative roles soon become very difficult to distinguish from other bureaucrats.

It is conceivable that the self-regulatory process might be more sensitive to the nuances of quality of care than an external alternative; but to the extent that the infinite variety of the clinical environment is used as an excuse for 'business as usual' and lip service to collective control, the whole strategy will be a failure (except, of course, as a delaying tactic). And if autonomy *per se* is as much of an objective in its own right as it is a putative contributor to patient outcomes, then it really does not matter if the standards enforced by physicians collectively might be somewhat different from those which might be enforced by governments or private payers. Clinical freedom, for the bulk of the profession, is equally threatened, either way.

That is not to say that the average clinician, if he/she *had* to sacrifice a substantial degree of clinical freedom, would not prefer to be monitored and directed by his/her peers, rather than the ultimate indignity of 'lay control'. But the central question then is, how serious is the external threat? Before circling the wagons under the direction of Wennberg and Brook, physicians might reasonably want to know how many Indians are really out there, and what the chances are of fighting them off in the traditional manner, without any significant sacrifice of the right to practise as one pleases. Are the times really changing, in such a way as to require this radical shift in individual and collective health policy?

It is worth noting two things. First, the most articulate advocates of the external threat are working in the USA, which is very much the odd man out in its arrangements for the organisation and funding of health care, compared with the other countries of the developed world (Abel-Smith, 1985; Scheiber and Poullier, 1988). The instability of such arrangements in the USA, compared with virtually everywhere else, is a consequence not only of that country's size and diversity, but also of its complete failure to discover a set of arrangements capable of placing any upper limit on the share of national resources which it devotes to health care. Those approaches used successfully in other nations are unacceptable for ideological reasons. Consequently, the American environment remains dynamically unstable. Large changes in institutional structures have occurred in the last decade, and it seems inevitable, from the on-going cost experience, that they will continue. Second, the American enthusiasm for or fear of structural change was most prominent in the early 1980s, during the introduction of the federal Prospective Payment System (DRGs) for hospitals, and the rapid spread of managed care plans, Health Maintenance Organizations and Preferred Provider Organizations, which were predicted to transform the power structure of health care delivery. Five years later, it appears that these expectations were somewhat overheated (Weiner *et al.*, 1987; Gabel *et al.*, 1988; Ginzburg, 1988). Surprisingly little change has occurred beneath the shift in organisational forms.

There certainly have been some substantial erosions of physician autonomy in particular settings, but it is hard to get an overall picture. However, the very fact that the cost escalation in the USA continues unabated suggests that the 'revolution' is not yet over. The real changes in health care organisation may be just beginning (Amara *et al.*, 1988). On the other hand, the intellectual tradition which advocates responding to cost increases by passing them on to someone else rather than trying to contain them is still alive and well in the USA (Manning *et al.*, 1987). So long as this line of debate can be sustained, it will help to block any effective action (Evans, 1988b).

Thus, an American physician might very well conclude that 'business as usual' was quite sustainable for a number of years yet, and hang the variations. In any case, the revolution does not have to be held off forever, only until the current leadership of the profession have finished their careers. *Le deluge, s'il y sera, aprés moi.*

Outside the USA the picture is entirely different, despite the similarity of rhetoric. Providers claim underfunding, and perceive grave threats to the quality of care in every attempt to restrict their resources and professional ambitions. Governments and quasi-public payment agencies allege cost explosions and an inability to pay more in the straitened circumstances of the 1980s. But behind the simultaneous cost explosions and institutional starvation, most nations in the developed world have stabilised the share of their resources which they devote to health care. Consequently, unlike the USA, their institutions for organisation and payment are also relatively stable. Revolutions are not in process, or on the horizon, because the existing institutions work (Note 17).

They do not work perfectly, by a very long shot. There is plenty of readily identifiable room for improvement, as, indeed, the widespread evidence of practice variations indicates. On the other hand, the fact that such variations *are* found universally, and are not just a feature of certain modes of organisation and reimbursement (Vayda, 1973; McPherson *et al.*, 1982), indicates that they are very deep-rooted in the structure of medical practice. It suggests that they are a characteristic of the culture and technology of medicine, which is common across national boundaries.

This in turn implies that any attempt to smooth out such variations by organisational reform will at least have to develop structures which are significantly different from any currently in place in the developed world. As noted above, this is, in fact, exactly what Enthoven (1988a, b) recommends. The increasingly apparent inadequacy of current American arrangements, and their inability to accept the ideological implications of others' experience, may eventually result in that country developing a unique alternative system, based primarily in the private sector, which could conceivably be more successful than the predominantly public systems in operation in the rest of the developed world (Rodwin, 1987). However, the experience of the last decade provides no grounds for optimism in the near term.

In this context, physicians outside, or even in, the USA might very well reject the call to 'circle the wagons'. They might, rather, conclude that, whatever the implications of variations in medical practice, it would be premature to give up their autonomy in self-defence against external threats which might not materialise, and in any case might be fought off by more traditional means. The organisational changes which would be required before any serious external threat to autonomy was likely to be mounted, are probably greater than is politically feasible outside the USA.

On the other hand, by taking collective action to deal with such variations, physicians would lend legitimacy to the concerns of those who view them with alarm, and would create institutions which might at a later date be influenced or even taken over by others. After all, if practice variations are such a serious matter that physicians themselves are trying to take corrective action, and if it turns out that action is ineffective – the variations persist – might not others outside the profession offer to lend a hand? Better to let sleeping, or even half-awake, dogs lie.

The soundness of this policy depends critically on providers' predictions as to the likely response of payers. Will these 'outsiders' seize on variations in practice patterns as an excuse to attack clinical freedom in the pursuit of cost containment, as feared by Brook *et al.* and hoped by the *Economist*? Well, they have shown no sign of doing so for the last 20 years. Are the times changing? Perhaps. But so far it appears that the major interest in practice patterns has come from reimbursers who are *not* in a position to do anything serious about them. Those governments and government-backed reimbursement agencies with real power and authority to intervene have stayed well away from practice patterns. This is probably not accidental.

FIRST MAN OVER THE BARRICADE GETS THE SPEAR THROUGH THE CHEST

Consider the position of a (public or private) agency responsible for reimbursing health care providers. In most countries of the developed world, that agency has evolved an on-going relationship with the providers of care which is a combination of conflict and co-operation. After all, bureaucrats cannot themselves deliver care. On the other hand, real life patients (outside the economics textbooks) cannot pay for very much of it. The relationship with providers is an on-going struggle for advantage, but neither could get along without the other.

The political pressures on such an agency are to maintain an adequate balance between access to care, quality of care and cost containment. In this balance, public perceptions are critical. On the other side of the table, providers are interested in access to care, quality of care and cost expansion. (From time to time they may allege a public-spirited interest in cost containment, but anyone believing this has fairies at the bottom of the garden.)

Both sides are genuinely interested in the welfare of the public which they both serve in different ways: providers do not really want to supply harmful or useless care, any more than reimbursers want to pay for it. And reimbursers do not really want to restrict the availability of genuinely effective care; they do, however, have to maintain some control over total outlays.

Now the agency is confronted with the practice variations evidence, which implies that a considerable amount of the care being provided is probably not justified by the patient's condition. What should the agency do? If it launches an attempt to save money by discouraging 'unnecessary' care, it will instantly be accused of 'practising medicine' (Note 18). By attacking the citadel of professional autonomy, it will guarantee a bitter political battle. It will be opposed not only by organised medicine, but also by the majority of individual practitioners, who are, in the main, still accepted by most of the public as 'the experts' in specifically clinical matters.

Who will be its allies in such a battle? Not the epidemiologists; they have already made it clear that they regard their research findings as a justification for redeployment of effort by the medical community, not for cost-cutting. And they have been equally clear that these matters are best left to the professionals to work out among themselves. The agency will find its actions labelled as 'ill-informed and dangerous' (Chassin *et al.*, 1986). When the political arguments begin over the proper interpretation of the variations literature, its authors will be lined up with the providers, not the cost-cutters.

But surely those who pay for care – taxpayers, premium-payers, employers and unions, more generally the community in its role as payer for, rather than receiver of, services – will they not be strong supporters? At the very least, the Minister of Finance, or his equivalent? Well, no, probably not.

As noted above, every developed country outside the USA has discovered that it is possible to limit the growth of health care costs, to at least a roughly constant share of national income, *without* probing into what providers actually do with those resources. A combination of fee negotiation, price control and global budgeting – a collection of public administrative mechanisms – has been used in different ways to contain overall spending (Evans, 1986, 1988b).

Culyer (1988) suggests that to the economist's traditional consideration of controls over 'demand' for and 'supply' of health care (terms which definitely do *not* have their usual textbook meaning when applied in this setting) must be added direct control over finance – total outlays. One way or another, countries have all used this direct limitation in addition to controls over supply and to a much lesser degree, if at all, demand.

The success of this control process, despite its political costs, indicates that intervention in the specifics of clinical practice is not a necessary condition for cost containment. And there is no reason to believe that a more rational approach to medical practice would be a sufficient condition either. As noted above, its most enthusiastic advocates are distinctly ambiguous on this point.

More generally, while we have heretofore postulated the provision of 'effective' care as the objective which, in principle, unites patients, providers and payers alike, in fact the situation is not that simple. In any given clinical situation, it may be possible to define the boundaries between the care that is 'needed' according to prevailing clinical standards and that which is not. But for the community as a whole, it is probably impossible to determine any level of provision beyond which no one's health could be improved by any conceivable additional services. Furthermore, as emerges *inter alia* from the variations litera- ture, clinical standards are themselves malleable, and shift with the availability of resources. When more is available, more will be (defined by the experts as) needed. Thus, there is a grain of truth behind the position of those who reject the relevance of the concept of need – at least while they are themselves healthy.

If 'needs', in a technical sense, are indefinitely expansible, and all can never be met, it follows that, as Williams (1978) has emphasised, expert judgements of 'need' can never be used as a basis for determining the overall level of allocation of community resources to health care. The experts *qua* experts will always demand more, on the basis of perceived unmet need. It is up to the general citizenry, or their elected representa- tives, to decide when enough is enough.

The logic of this position is impeccable and its predictive power is not bad either. But that will be of little comfort to our embattled agency, venturing into the practice of medicine at second-hand, armed with a stack of computer print-outs and a collection of academic articles whose authors repudiate its efforts. To the extent that it *does* succeed in discouraging certain excessive rates of activity in certain regions or by certain practitioners, it can confidently predict that any resources thus freed will be absorbed in other forms of care provision – meeting other needs and, not incidentally, maintaining providers' incomes. (This has also been the fate of resources 'saved' by technical innovations in care which have genuinely reduced the resources required – most recently the lithotripter, earlier the CT scanner.) To prevent this reabsorption will require yet another battle.

Indeed, there is even worse news on the horizon. The advocates of cost control through practice standards (including this one) have always assumed that unexplained high rates of servicing represent correspond- ing high rates of 'unnecessary' servicing, and conversely for low rates. It was presumed that if and when detailed and thorough studies of outcomes were done, this would be confirmed (recall Webber and Goldbeck, or McClure and Shaller). A recent, very thorough study *has* been done in the USA, not, admittedly, of outcomes, but of the appropriateness of use of several common procedures – coronary angiography, carotid endarterectomy and upper GI tract endoscopy – by expert panel review of patient charts (Chassin et al., 1987). The findings are somewhat paradoxical.

The study found substantial rates of inappropriate use – 17% of all angiographies and GI endoscopies, and 32% of endarterectomies, according to the experts' judgements. Moreover, the study data were for 1981, and rates have since increased, suggesting that if the same criteria were applied today, even higher rates of inappropriate use would be found. So far so good; plenty of scope for cost savings through more appropriate practice patterns.

The bad news, however, is that the study examined rates of inappropriate use in previously identified areas of high, average and low use of such procedures, and found no systematic differences among them.

'. . . we did not find evidence to support the hypothesis that areas with high use of medical and surgical procedures show these high rates primarily or to any meaningful extent because physicians in these areas perform these procedures more often for inappropriate indications . . .' [p. 2535–6].

Absence of evidence is not, of course, evidence of absence. Peer judgements are not the same as outcomes. The study was of only three procedures, in three areas. And it certainly showed evidence, on the most conservative of criteria, of substantial overservicing and waste. But it does *not* show that one can safely infer relative rates of unnecessary use, across regions, from relative rates of use. Its findings are thus powerful ammunition to attack anyone who adopts an explicit policy of attempting to equalise regional rates of use of specific procedures. Our hypothetical payment agency could expect to hear a good deal about this study.

WHOSE SIDE AM I SUPPOSED TO BE ON?

All in all, it would probably not be surprising if our payment agency, having worked out the costs and benefits, also decided to let sleeping dogs lie. Providers, putting themselves in the payers' shoes, may predict such behaviour, which in turn will discourage them from taking action. So long as payers can maintain a politically acceptable level of (perceived) access, providers can protect their professional autonomy, and both can live with the resulting amount of expenditures/incomes, the institutional structure would appear to be quite stable.

Of course, the rhetoric gets quite heated. Representatives of both sides of this relationship must assure their respective constituencies that they are vigilant and energetic in their struggle for higher/lower costs and greater/lesser efficiency/accountability. Moreover, they play out their on-going struggle in front of an audience of patients, taxpayers and voters whose support must be retained. In this perpetual contest over fees, budgets and new investments, it is possible that the variations data might be presented to the public (as they certainly could be!) to rebut professional claims that cost containment was a threat to health. But that is quite different from a serious policy to deal with the variations themselves.

Thus, the failure of payers to respond to the information from variations data can be summarised as: 'Too dangerous, and anyway we can achieve our critical objectives by other means.' From the providers' side: 'We ourselves do not find variations a problem, and we do not find the external threat credible.'

Alternative interpretations, of course, exist. One, emphasised by the *Economist* (1988), is that the databases available to payers have not in the past been sufficient to support (or defend) intervention. But now, in the USA at least, '. . . mega-databases will collect the masses of information contained in the medical records of insurance companies. . . . The health of patients will be monitored . . .', *etc*. The times are changing, because the information technology is changing.

Unfortunately for this view, 'mega-databases' have been available in Canada for decades. As far back as 1974, the federal Deputy Minister of Health pointed out that the key problem was not collecting more data, but figuring out what to do with them. Canadian provincial governments, with both powerful incentives and some authority to contain costs, have on the whole made a fairly decent job of it (Evans, 1986; Culyer, 1988; Evans *et al.*, 1989b). But they have not done so by getting into the details of medical practice, and that has not been because of lack of data (Note 19). They chose not to.

They chose not to, apparently, for very good political reasons. Yet the implications of the practice variations data remain. They represent strong *prima facie* evidence of inappropriate servicing, waste of resources and possibly actual harm to patients. The problem is that it has not been in the interests of either providers or payers to do anything about it. Despite their expressed and probably genuine mutual interest in the welfare of patients and the effectiveness of care, and the interest of payers at least in efficiency and cost containment, the constellation of forces and objectives in which they interact leads to stalemate.

THE TIMES ARE ALWAYS CHANGING – BUT HOW?

The question, then, is what changes are under way, or possible, which might break the stalemate? The various possibilities offered seem to fall into three classes: (1) greater public involvement, (2) organisational restructuring and (3) increasing pressure on overall health resources.

(1) Costs of inappropriate servicing are borne by the public, as both patients and, eventually, payers. If neither of the agents responsible for acting on their behalf is willing or able to deal with the situation, perhaps the answer is to get the public more involved. This could occur in two ways. Individual patients could become more informed and involved in the treatment decision, and the public collectively, the electorate, could be made more aware of the range of, and flimsy justification for, current patterns of treatment.

On the first point, a great deal of nonsense has been talked about the increase in consumerism and the possibilities of patients taking over the management of their own care, usually by people with an ideological commitment to the marketplace who hope that wishing will make it so (e.g. the *Economist*, 1988). The reality is that an increasing proportion of medical and hospital care is provided to elderly patients, in conditions of diminished capacity (e.g. Barer *et al.*, 1987, 1988b; Evans *et al.*, 1989a). At the same time, the increasing complexity of care is making it more, not less, difficult for patients to have an effective voice.

The provision of more information to, and ensuring of more auton-omy for, patients is surely to be applauded and assisted, for a number of reasons. But there is no evidence to show that this has had a significant effect on the appropriateness of medical practice in the past, or reason to believe that it will in the future. Where, after all, do most patients get their medical advice? Patients undergo unnecessary procedures, firmly believing that they are necessary, because they are told so by physicians who also believe so and whom they trust. Unless this relationship is changed, and it is by no means clear that it should be, the individual patient is unlikely to be a major source of pressure to rationalise practice patterns.

The possibility of informing the public at large – voters and taxpayers, rather than patients – is more interesting, although such initiatives have as yet had little effect. The Health Care Financing Administration in the USA has published case-mix adjusted mortality rates for different hospitals, while the *Los Angeles Times* (Steinbrook, 1988) has published comparative data on (wide variations in) surgical mortality for five common procedures in selected California hospitals. The former has received intense criticism of both the data and the fact of publication; there is no evidence of patient response (Vladeck *et al.*, 1988).

However, patient-based mortality rates are relatively easy for the general public to understand, even if they may be misinterpreted. Population-based procedural rates are substantially more difficult to interpret, much less to act upon. However, in 1970 the Government of Manitoba published some quite extraordinary information on regional variations in rates of particular surgical procedures. The response from the medical profession was violently negative; from the public at large, virtually nil.

It may be that the significance of the practice variations literature can be communicated to the general public, but this would certainly require much more than the broader dissemination of research results in their usual form. It would require a focused information campaign, with objectives clearly specified in advance. Some sort of behavioural response would obviously be sought; we shall return to this below.

(2) 'Organisational restructuring' covers a multitude of possibilities. As one example, Enthoven (1988a, b) advocates the creation or recognition of 'sponsors' – organisations taking responsibility for a defined population such as an employee group and their dependents. The sponsor would then oversee the contracting between group members and competitive suppliers of health care, who would bid for the members on a capitation basis. The sponsor and the individual members would each have some financial involvement in the choice. Sponsors would then have an incentive, and the resources, to investigate the practice patterns of the competing medical care suppliers. They would identify for their members providers whose practice patterns were overly costly, or even strike outliers from their list of approved plans.

There are a number of problems with such a proposal, particularly in a competitive environment, and sponsors might very well find it more profitable and less difficult to weed out high-cost patients than to try to manage medical care at arm's length (Evans, 1988a). But Enthoven's proposal does attempt to create new policy makers, who might assemble and act upon information about practice variations in order to contain costs as well as to improve quality of care.

Similar possibilities arise in other systems. Regional and district managers in the National Health Service of the UK, non-clinicians assigned fixed budgets with which to 'purchase' care for their populations, and judged according to the outcomes achieved, might very well have an interest in practice variations. Their goal would presumably be the more effective deployment of externally determined resources rather than the cost containment which is central to Enthoven's proposal. But they represent new sources of policy, with new objectives.

Yet another variant on this theme has been suggested in Canada (Ontario, 1974; Evans, 1988c). One could modify the present fee-for-service system for reimbursing physicians, by introducing regional fixed budgets based on, *inter alia*, the size and age–sex structure of the regional population. These would then be available to reimburse the care of members of that population, wherever received. If fee claims submitted on behalf of a region's population exceeded or fell short of the budgetary allowance, they would be uniformly discounted or supplemented by the proportion necessary to achieve equality.

The regional budgets could be divided by type of service (general practice, specialty, diagnostic) and linked to hospital utilisation and costs, in such a way that physicians' fees in each region were affected by their choice of practice style. This would encourage physicians to co-ordinate their behaviour, and to evaluate each other's practice patterns, by making each region similar to a geographically based, capitated Health Maintenance Organisation. The new source of policy, with new incentives, under this system would be the regional medical community, more or less formally organised.

Regional budgeting leaves the control of practice patterns in the hands of the medical community, and does not introduce other entities intruding upon their autonomy. On the other hand, it places physicians collectively at economic risk for their differences in practice style. Variations in practice patterns become costs to (or rewards for) other physicians, rather than payers or patients.

(3) Finally, the most commonly identified force acting to encourage greater attention to variations in medical practice is the 'spiralling cost of health care' (Note 20). The logical connection appears simple: rising costs pressing on limited resources will require greater attention to efficiency and effectiveness; hence, to the relationship between needs and services. Inevitably, payers and providers alike will have to find ways of rationalising patterns of care.

As usual, the simple analysis is wrong on both facts and logic. It neglects the fundamental conflict of interest between payers and providers, which is expressed in the ambiguity of the phrase 'cost control'. Both parties do indeed want to control costs, but they want to move them in different directions. They *cannot* co-operate on this issue, with the best will in the world.

The confusion arises from a tendency, politically understandable, to try to portray the 'pressure of rising costs' as a force external to the health care system, like gravity or the tides. The factors usually pointed to are demographic changes, technology and 'public expectations'.

In fact, however, a number of analyses of demographic change have shown that these do not account for more than a small proportion of recent increases in health costs, and are unlikely to do so in the foreseeable future. The major sources of cost pressure are changes in how people in particular circumstances are cared for – the increasing intensity of servicing (Evans, 1985; Barer *et al.*, 1987).

Nor can one argue that increasing servicing intensity and cost are simply a response to changing technology and/or public expectations.

At this point the evidence on effectiveness of care becomes relevant, *inter alia* that on variations in medical practice. It is simply *not true* that patterns of care, and cost, are determined by the needs of patients; that is what this book is about. How, then, can one claim with a straight face that the redefinitions of need emerging from the evolution of technology *require* increases in resources? (Note 21)

Yet the argument that health care is 'underfunded' continues to be urged by providers in every developed country outside the USA. Even in the USA the rhetoric of constrained resources is commonplace – as Reinhardt (1987) points out, a complete divorce of rhetoric from reality. The claims of demographic doom and technological determinism are untouched by the accumulation of counter-evidence, indicating that evidence is simply irrelevant to the issue. The need for more resources is not a conclusion, but an axiom.

To the extent, then, that cost pressures in the health care system are pressures for increased incomes, coming from a rapidly growing number of providers, with increasing technological ambitions, backed by an equally ambitious pharmaceutical and equipment industry looking for new markets, that pressure will in no way be abated by rationalisation of patterns of care. Even if 'bigger and better' epidemiological studies result in the unambiguous identification of unnecessary services, and providers can be induced to discontinue them, the result will simply be a shift into other activities. The alternative, of course, would be a fall in provider incomes; fortunately, there are always unmet needs (Note 22).

The 'internal/external' balance of cost pressures is, of course, open to debate. However, the point to grasp is that the assumption that increasing cost pressures will have any bearing on policy towards medical practice variations requires that one also assumes that those pressures are external to the health care system. For example, a payment agency which interprets its expenditures as primarily determined by the numbers and income expectations of the physicians it is responsible for reimbursing will obviously not expect careful attention to practice variations to mitigate any financial pressures it faces.

However, there may be another possibility. Providers of care routinely place political pressure on payers through the claim of 'your money or your life'. Cost containment, it is alleged, leads to 'underfunding' – unmet needs, suffering, even preventable deaths. But this claim, as emphasised above, rests on the assumption that servicing patterns and costs are in fact closely linked to needs, precisely the assumption which is undermined by the practice variations literature. Might not a payment agency respond to provider pressure for 'more' by going public with these data?

Such a campaign would have quite different objectives from those of our hapless agency above, which we suggested would find itself in an unwinnable battle over professional autonomy. It would have the narrower goal, not of actually changing practice patterns (still less of moderating costs thereby), but of discrediting or at least blunting the 'your money or your life' claim, in the eyes of the electorate. 'Do not ask for more resources, until you can show that you are making effective use of those you already have.' The intended audience would be the electorate, not providers.

This would risk a substantial escalation in the on-going conflict between providers and payers, because it would represent a direct attack on the public credibility of providers. Of course, 'your money or your life' represents an attempt to put that credibility into play for economic objectives, in a way which the variations literature, along with other forms of evidence, shows to be unjustifiable. The rejection of provider priorities and claims is implicit in any conflict over the resources to be allocated to health care, other than a completely passive policy of signing blank cheques. But a deliberate focus on medical practice variations calls explicitly into question the clinical behaviour of individual practitioners.

Providers collectively might choose to take a more serious interest in practice variations, in order to defuse the argument. However, they are more likely, for reasons outlined above, to react with violent denials of the validity of both the data and the whole question. In such a confrontational context, the prospects for a detached and scientific assessment of the implications of practice variations for the quality of medical care are rather small.

Given the potentially explosive nature of the issue, it is not surprising that so many researchers in this field have emphasised that the evidence be used only 'to help doctors become better doctors'. Nor is this an unworthy aim. The redeployment of resources away from ineffective activities, even if it is only towards as yet unevaluated ones, is probably on balance an improvement.

By taking the variations issue away from the cost-cutters, however, and down-playing its implication of wasted resources in the absence of external accountability, they substantially weaken its prospects for policy attention. There is a very large crowd of people with proposals for 'improving the quality of health care'. Most also claim that they will add little or nothing to health costs, or at least whatever they add will be matched by savings somewhere else. (Someone else's income will fall, or job disappear.) When pressed for details, they reply that surely the really important issue is quality of care.

The cost-cutters will not, of course, go away, and they will continue to interpret the variations evidence as supportive of their activities. As indeed they should, if the proper decision rule is 'when in doubt, don't'. 'When in doubt, do' makes the most sense if one is *selling* services, not buying them (Note 23). But more formalised and targeted policy responses will require prospects of larger payoffs than yet another unmeasurable improvement in 'quality of care'. Unless and until research and researchers on practice variations begin to offer ways of relieving the endless pressure for more health spending, the dog is likely to remain quite quiet. Sensible dogs wait for real bones.

NOTES

[1] In the late 1960s and early 1970s the Management and Operations Research Unit of the Ontario Hospital Services Commission reported directly to the Chairman of the Commission, and provided very detailed data on the differences in patterns of care among different hospitals and across regions within the province. The policy response was to disband the Unit. . . .

[2] In the discussion we follow Lomas (1989) in using 'health policy' to refer to the policies not only of governments and their agents – 'public' policies – but also those of quasi-public or wholly private entities such as insurers, hospitals, medical associations and individual clinicians.

[3] There are several other views of health care, arising from different branches of the social sciences. The most serious alternative contender comes from economics, and posits that in fact health care can be adequately represented as essentially similar to the hypothetical standard commodity of the textbooks, purchased by 'consumers' for reasons best known to themselves. The utilisation of this commodity is then described within the standard textbook intellectual framework, without any essential role for the concepts of 'health', or 'needs', or 'professions'.

However, this approach has not been particularly successful in explaining the very peculiar institutional structure of the health care industry, in every developed country (Culyer, 1982; Evans, 1983, 1984). Nor have its policy recommendations received serious attention (except when they happened to coincide with and further the objectives of established interest groups within the health care industry), largely because they rest on (non-articulated, but fundamental) value bases which are not widely accepted in developed societies. Its adherents are primarily restricted to economists in the USA, and a handful of their overseas intellectual colonies.

[4] This approach does not commit one to a definition of health as 'merely the absence of disease or injury'; it does, however, define the health *care* system in relatively narrow terms. But if one takes a broad, WHO-style definition of health, and at the same time takes cognisance of *all* the factors which can affect health in that sense, there are few if any activities which are *not* part of the health care system! Concepts with no exclusions are not particularly helpful.

[5] This is not to suggest that the social constructs of professionalisation and not-for-profit organisation are always or completely successful in protecting the interests of patients against those of providers. But if they have *no* influence on provider behaviour, and yield *no* benefits for patients over and above what would emerge in an ordinary, arm's-length, *caveat emptor* marketplace, then it is hard to see any other justification for their continued existence.

[6] 'Appropriate care' is defined in terms of reasonable expectation of benefit. No one is perfect; the care may turn out badly for a number of reasons. But the interventions offered should be more likely to do more good than harm, based on the state of knowledge which the provider might reasonably be expected to possess. There is obviously a great deal of room for interpretation in practice, but the basic principle is clear enough.

[7] In particular, even if one has decided which services are 'needed', there remains the question of their cost. This in turn is determined by both the efficiency with which services are provided and the relative incomes of providers of care. The interests of providers and of payers are not congruent on these points.

[8] In fact, experimental data cannot absolutely eliminate this possibility either; they merely reduce the probability of such confounding effects to a lower level.

[9] One begins by assuming, implicitly, that the provision of care is always and everywhere determined by the needs of the patient, so that variations in care are therefore simply evidence of differences in needs. The failure to find any direct evidence of such 'differences in needs', or any plausible correlate which would explain the differences in care patterns, means that the investigator did not look hard enough. This form of argument has been well developed by tobacco companies, anti-fluoridationists, and neoclassical economists; but it does not, and is not meant to, lead towards enlightenment.

[10] One might argue that the clinical community has simply taken an appropriately skeptical 'wait-and-see' attitude towards findings which were, initially at least, susceptible to different interpretations. To this there are two responses. First, the assumption that the *status quo* is satisfactory until the alternative is proven beyond all reasonable doubt represents a location of the burden of proof for which there is no methodological justification. The *prima facie* evidence 20 years ago indicated that practice patterns could not be justified on the basis of underlying population needs. Ignoring this evidence was itself an implicit policy. Second, the clinical community has never had any difficulty in responding to new technologies in the absence of proof of effectiveness – quite the contrary. The clinical policy decision rules are quite clearly asymmetric.

[11] Buck's view that studies are *impossible* without clinical support may be too strong. It is certainly possible to derive detailed information on patterns of physician practice from modern data collection systems, without the consent or co-operation of clinicians. However, the *interpretation* of those variations, at least through the process of large-scale peer audit which he describes, certainly depends upon clinician co-operation.

[12] Webber and Goldbeck (1984: p. 69) claim that there is 'growing understanding that UR [utilisation review] is in the long-term interests of the fee-for-service physician community', but it is unclear what meaning they attach to the statement. The context suggests that they may be offering UR as the lesser of two evils: Rationalise and control your own utilisation patterns, even if that means lower incomes, or be driven out of the market entirely (or absorbed) by the non-fee-for-service, 'managed care' plans.

[13] The failure of the 'marketplace' philosophy and policy to contain total costs in the USA will presumably give rise to another wave of policy, and a new challenge to physicians, but it is still too early to see what that will be (Gabel *et*

al., 1988). Amara *et al.* (1988) predict a major shift from 'shallow' to 'deep' capitation, arguing that the structural changes in the USA have so far been more shadow than substance, and that the real competitive revolution is yet to come. If *that* does not work, is there anything left but national health insurance?

[14]Of course, the commitment to autonomy for its own sake also admits an economic dimension. One does not need to be a highly trained chef to read a cookbook. Some skills are certainly required, but they are nowhere near as extensive, or costly, as those required to invent new dishes from scratch. To the extent that clinical practice is systematised in standards and protocols, it will become increasingly difficult to suppress competitors with intermediate level skills who can do the same work at lower cost, and quite possibly with better outcomes.

[15]Medicine is often described as an art, rather than or as well as a science. But art evolves; it does not progress. Medicine claims to progress, and most of us believe the claim. If medicine were really an art, there would be no more justification for licensing its practitioners, and suppressing their competitors, than there is for licensing artists. Too often, it appears that spokesmen for professions emphasise their scientific basis when they are seeking favours from the state – regulations or subsidies – and emphasise their art when they are asked to account for results.

[16]The experience of Wolfe and Detmer (1984) is instructive. They studied variations in total and ancillary charges, and in lengths of stay, for two procedures (routine inguinal hernia and uncomplicated appendicectomy), performed by attending surgeons and house officers in a single hospital. Large differences in average costs per patient were found for different clinicians, after standardisation for patient characteristics. When the results were presented to the clinicians involved, their first reaction was to question the validity of the data. 'Only when they were assured that one of their colleagues had personally reviewed all of the records ... did they begin to seriously examine [sic] the resultant data' [p. 17].

Moreover, Wolfe and Detmer did not call into question the appropriateness of the surgical procedures themselves, as is implicitly or explicitly done in the bulk of the practice variations literature. The potential savings indicated by their findings would, if they materialised, reduce only the incomes of salaried hospital staff, not those of the surgeons.

[17]Indeed, the growing sense of dissatisfaction with these institutions among providers is attributable precisely to the fact that they *do* work. They succeed in imposing an external constraint on the appetite of the health care system for ever more resources. There appear to be no *internal* limits on that appetite, and no natural constraints on what can be defined as 'needs', so friction between the providers of care and those responsible for protecting the resources of the rest of society is inevitable (Evans, 1988b).

In Canada, for example, the representatives of organised medicine routinely predict the 'collapse' of the country's universal health insurance plans, unless they receive more money. Their preferred alternative, since bargaining with provincial governments over fee levels has turned out to be surprisingly tough (Barer *et al.*, 1988a), is to regain the right to bill patients directly, over and above the public fee schedules. This, they allege, will control the costs of health care by 'deterring' unnecessary use, and at the same time will increase the flow of funds into the health care system and relieve its 'underfunding'.

Obviously, only one of these allegations can be true; the evidence (as well as the assumption of enlightened self-interest) suggests that it is the latter. Extra-billing will relieve the underfunding of physicians' incomes. The connection between the perceived adequacy of funding for health care and the income aspirations of physicians has also been emphasised by Reinhardt (1987).

[18] Unless, of course, it does so by imposing, or permitting physicians to impose, additional charges upon patients, in which case its activities will be applauded. An elementary application of the assumption of enlightened self-interest indicates that such a policy will threaten neither providers' autonomy nor their incomes; experience supports this expectation.

[19] The data available to Canadian provincial governments have many shortcomings. But to the extent that they are inadequate, this is by the deliberate choice of the government involved. They have always had ample authority to improve their databases if they chose. As a result, the quality and usefulness of the health system data are very variable from one province to another. But the constraint has been political will.

[20] Health care costs always spiral, although no one, to my knowledge, has ever tried to represent their behaviour in polar coordinates.

[21] The technology assessment literature is also relevant here (e.g. Banta *et al.*, 1981; Guyatt *et al.*, 1986), emphasising the weak connection between the introduction and spread of a new technology and its demonstrated effectiveness.

[22] This is a critical point. Obviously clinicians learn, and their activities do change. The dramatic reduction in tonsillectomy rates is an example, although also one which shows an extraordinarily slow response to overwhelming evidence. (It may be that, in this case, the believers simply had to retire or die, and be replaced with a generation trained differently.) Where there is unambiguous evidence that a procedure is useless, and particularly if it is actually harmful, its performance will decline. But the resources thus freed, whether professional time, operating rooms, hospital beds, or whatever, are not withdrawn from service. Something else is done, and paid for, instead.

[23] As prudent purchasers on behalf of the rest of the community, payers' attempts to contain costs are no less worthy than providers' concerns for 'quality' – and a good deal more specific.

REFERENCES

Abel-Smith, B. (1985). Who is the odd man out?: The experience of Western Europe in containing the costs of health care. *Milbank Memorial Fund Quarterly/ Health and Society*, **63**(1), 1–17

Amara, R., Morrison, J. I. and Schmid, G. (1988). *Looking Ahead at American Health Care*. McGraw-Hill Healthcare Information Center, Washington, D.C.

Banta, H. D., Behney, C. and Willems, J. S. (1981). *Toward Rational Technology in Medicine: Considerations for Health Policy*. Springer, New York

Barer, M. L., Evans, R. G., Hertzman, C. and Lomas, J. (1987). Aging and health care utilisation: new evidence on old fallacies. *Social Science and Medicine*, **24**(10), 851–62

Barer, M. L., Evans, R. G. and Labelle, R. J. (1988a). Fee controls as cost control: tales from the frozen North. *Milbank Quarterly*, **66**(1), 1–64

Barer, M. L., Pulcins, I. R., Evans, R. G. *et al.* (1988b). Diagnosing senescence: the medicalization of B.C.'s elderly. Health Policy Research Unit Discussion Paper 88(6), July, University of British Columbia, Vancouver, B.C.

Bock, R. S. (1988). The pressure to keep prices high at a walk-in clinic. *New England Journal of Medicine*, **319**(12) 785–7

Bowen, O. E. (1987). Shattuck Lecture – What is quality care? *New England Journal of Medicine*, **316**(25), 1578–80

Brook, R. H., Lohr, K. N., Chassin, M. *et al.* (1984). Geographic variations in the use of services: do they have any clinical significance? *Health Affairs*, **3**(2), 63–73

Buck, N. (1988). Regional and district variations in perioperative deaths. In Ham, C. (Ed.), *Health Care Variations: Assessing the Evidence*. Research Report No. 2, The King's Fund Institute, London, pp. 27–9

Bunker, J. P. (1970). Surgical manpower. A comparison of operations and surgeons in the United States and in England and Wales. *New England Journal of Medicine*, **282**(3), 135–44

Chassin, M. R., Brook, R. H., Park, R. E. *et al.* (1986). Variations in the use of medical and surgical services by the Medicare population. *New England Journal of Medicine*, **314**(5), 285–90

Chassin, M., Kosecoff, J., Winslow, C. M. *et al.* (1987). Does inappropriate use explain geographic variations in the use of health care services? *Journal of the American Medical Association*, **258**(18), 2533–7

Copenhagen Collaborating Center (1987). *Bibliography on Regional Variations in Health Care, Number 2: 1987*. World Health Organization Regional Office for Europe, Copenhagen

Culyer, A. J. (1982). The NHS and the market: Images and realities. In McLachlan, G. and Maynard, A. (Eds.), *The Public–Private Mix for Health: The Relevance and Effects of Change*. Nuffield Provincial Hospitals Trust, London, pp. 23–55

Culyer, A. J. (1988). *Health Expenditures in Canada: Myth and Reality, Past and Future*. Canadian Tax Foundation, Toronto

Economist (1988). Fallible doctors. Patient's dilemma. December 17, 19–21

Enthoven, A. C. (1985). *Reflections on the Management of the National Health Service*. The Nuffield Provincial Hospitals Trust (Occasional Papers No. 5), London

Enthoven, A. C. (1988a). Toward a model system for the financing and delivery of health care in the United States. In Leader, S. and Moon, M. (Eds.), *Changing America's Health Care System: Proposals for Legislative Action*, Scott Foresman, AARP Books, Glenview, Illnois, pp. 21–42

Enthoven, A. C. (1988b). *Theory and Practice of Managed Competition in Health Care Finance*. North-Holland, Amsterdam, pp. 75–118

Evans, R. G. (1983). The welfare economics of public health insurance: Theory and Canadian practice. In Soderstrom, L. (Ed.), *Social Insurance*. North-Holland, Amsterdam, pp. 71–104

Evans, R. G. (1984). *Strained Mercy: The Economics of Canadian Health Care*. Butterworths, Toronto

Evans, R. G. (1985). Illusions of necessity; evading responsibility for choice in health care. *Journal of Health Policy, Politics and Law*, **10**(3), 439–67

Evans, R. G. (1986). Finding the levers, finding the courage: Lessons from cost containment in North America. *Journal of Health Politics, Policy and Law,* **11**(4), 585–616

Evans, R. G. (1988a). Notes of a cat-skinner: alternative visions of the American system. In Leader, S. and Moon, M. (Eds.), *Changing America's Health Care System: Proposals for Legislative Action,* Scott Foresman, AARP Books, Glenview, Illinois, pp. 125–60

Evans, R. G. (1988b). Tension, compression, and shear: directions, stresses, and outcomes of health care cost control. Paper presented at the International Symposium on *Controlling Costs While Maintaining Health: The Experience of Canada, the United States of America, and the Federal Republic of Germany,* Bonn, FRG, June 27/28, 1988 (Health Policy Research Unit Discussion Paper **88**(13) (December), University of British Columbia, Vancouver, B.C.)

Evans, R. G. (1988c). Squaring the circle: reconciling fee-for-service with global expenditure control. Health Policy Research Unit Discussion Paper **88**(8) (August), University of British Columbia, Vancouver, B.C.

Evans, R. G., Barer, M. L., Hertzman, C. *et al.* (1989a). The long good-bye: the great transformation of the British Columbia hospital system. *Health Services Research,* October (forthcoming)

Evans, R. G., Lomas, J., Barer, M. L. *et al.* (1989b). Controlling health expenditure: the Canadian reality. *New England Journal of Medicine,* **320**(9), 571–7

Gabel, J., Jajich-Toth, C., de Lissovoy, G. *et al.* (1988). The changing world of group health insurance. *Health Affairs,* **7**(3), 48–65

Ginzburg, E. (1988). For-profit medicine. A reassessment. *New England Journal of Medicine,* **319**(12), 757–61

Guyatt, G., Feeny, D. and Tugwell, P. (Eds.) (1986). *Health Care Technology: Effectiveness, Efficiency, and Public Policy.* Institute for Research on Public Policy, Montreal

Ham, C. (Ed.) (1988). *Health Care Variations: Assessing the Evidence.* The King's Fund Institute (Research Report No. 2), London

Jennett, B. (1988). Variations data from surgeons, for surgeons. In Ham, C. (Ed.), *Health Care Variations: Assessing the Evidence.* The King's Fund Institute (Research Report No. 2), London, pp. 30–1

Lewis, C. E. (1969). Variations in the incidence of surgery. *New England Journal of Medicine,* **281**(16), 880–4

Lomas, J. and Barer, M. L. (1986). And who shall represent the public interest? The legacy of Canadian health manpower policy. In Evans, R. G. and Stoddart, G. L. (Eds.), *Medicare at Maturity: Achievements, Lessons and Challenges.* University of Calgary Press for the Banff Centre, Calgary, pp. 221–86

Lomas, J. (1989). Promoting clinical policy change: using the art to promote the science in medicine. This volume, pp. 174–91

Manning, W. G., Newhouse, J. P., Duan, N. *et al.* (1987). Health insurance and the demand for medical care. *American Economic Review,* **77**(3), 251–77

McClure, W. and Shaller, D. (1984). Variations in Medicare expenditure. *Health Affairs,* **3**(2), 120–9

McPherson, K., Wennberg, J. E., Hovind, O. B. and Clifford, P. (1982). Small area variations in the use of common surgical procedures: an international comparison of New England, England and Norway. *New England Journal of Medicine,* **307**(21), 1310–14

Ontario (1974). *Report of the Health Planning Task Force* (J. F. Mustard, chairman). Government of Ontario, Toronto

Paul-Shaheen, P., Clark, J. D. and Williams, D. (1987). Small area analysis: a review and analysis of the North American literature. *Journal of Health Politics, Policy and Law,* **12**(4), 741–809

Pearson, R. J. C., Smedby, B., Berfenstam, R. *et al.* (1968). Hospital caseloads in Liverpool, New England and Uppsala. *Lancet,* **2**, 559–66

Record, J. C. (Ed.) (1981). *Staffing Primary Care in 1990: Physician Replacement and Cost Savings.* Springer, New York

Reinhardt, U. E. (1987). Resource allocation in health care: the allocation of lifestyles to providers. *Milbank Quarterly,* **65**(2), 153–76

Renaud, M., Beauchemin, J., Lalonde, C. *et al.* (1980). Practice setting and prescribing profiles: the simulation of tension headaches to general practitioners working in different practice settings in the Montreal area. *American Journal of Public Health,* **70**(10), 1068–73

Rennels, G. D. and Shortliffe, E. H. (1987). Advanced computing for medicine. *Scientific American,* **257**(4), 154–61

Rodwin, V. G. (1987). American exceptionalism in the health sector: the advantages of 'backwardness' in learning from abroad. *Medical Care Review,* **44**(1), 119–54

Roos, N. P., Flowerdew, G., Wajda, A. and Tate, R. B. (1986). Variations in physicians' hospitalization practices: a population-based study in Manitoba, Canada. *American Journal of Public Health,* **76**(1), 45–51

Shapiro, M. (1978). *Getting Doctored.* Between the Lines, Kitchener, Ont.

Scheiber, G. and Poullier, J.-P. (1988). International health spending and utilization trends. *Health Affairs,* **7**(4), 105–12

Scovern, H. (1988). Hired help: a physician's experiences in a for-profit staff-model HMO. *New England Journal of Medicine,* **319**(12), 787–90

Spitzer, W. O. (1984). The nurse practitioner revisited: slow death of a good idea. *New England Journal of Medicine,* **310**(16), 1049–51

Starr, P. (1982). *The Social Transformation of American Medicine.* Basic Books, New York

Steinbrook, R. (1988). Hospital quality in California. *Health Affairs,* **7**(3), 235–6

Vayda, E. (1973). A comparison of surgical rates in Canada and in England and Wales. *New England Journal of Medicine,* **289**(23), 1224–9

Vladeck, B. C., Goodwin, E. J., Myers, L. P. and Sinisi, M. (1988). Consumers and hospitals: the HCFA 'death list'. *Health Affairs,* **7**(1), 122–5

Webber, A. and Goldbeck, W. B. (1984). Utilization Review. In Fox, P. D., Goldbeck, W. B. and Spies, J. J. (Eds.), *Health Care Cost Management: Private Sector Initiatives.* Health Administration Press, Ann Arbor, pp. 69–90

Weiner, S. L., Maxwell, J. H., Sapolsky, H. M. *et al.* (1987). Economic incentives and organizational realities: managing hospitals under DRGs. *Milbank Quarterly,* **65**(4), 463–87

Wennberg, J. E. (1984). Dealing with medical practice variations: a proposal for action. *Health Affairs,* **3**(2), 6–32

Wennberg, J. E. (1988). Practice variations and the need for outcomes research. In Ham, C. (Ed.), *Health Care Variations: Assessing the Evidence.* The King's Fund Institute (Research Report No. 2), London, pp. 32–5

Williams, A. (1978). Need: an economic exegesis. In Culyer, A. J. and Wright,

K. G. (Eds.), *Economic Aspects of Health Services*. Martin Robertson, London, pp. 32–45

Wolfe, B. L. and Detmer, D. (1984). The economics of surgical signatures. Discussion paper No. 212, Center for Health Economics and Law, University of Wisconsin, Madison, Wisconsin

CHAPTER 8

Variations from a Lay Perspective

Frede Vestergaard

What do patients – and potential patients, as we all are – expect from the health care system?

The answer is quite simple. We want a system which is at any time able to provide the best possible treatment, regardless of our ability to pay, personal position, etc. In Denmark and in most other European countries the claim is for equal access for equal need. The rich may have the right to buy a bigger and better car. But they do not have the right to better or preferential treatment.

This claim may not always be fulfilled. Private medicine, after all, does exist. But this is the principle to which doctors, health administrators and policy makers are expected to adhere. The best possible treatment (whatever that may be) is a citizen's right. The family doctor is expected to deliver this, if necessary by referring the patient on to a specialist or to hospital.

This process is based on a considerable amount of trust. The patient has to trust the family doctor and the doctors at the hospital. The individual patient does not as a rule know what is good for him. He will generally not be able to choose his own treatment; nonetheless he expects the best treatment available. He is then very dependent on his medical 'advisors', i.e. the doctors who are to treat him. He will have to trust that they can and do choose the appropriate treatment, as he will probably not be given any choice.

As the principle of medical treatment as a citizen's right is deeply entrenched in people's minds, most people, in Denmark at least, believe they are given the necessary treatment in so far as the doctor has been able to diagnose correctly. And they are probably right. However, we are now told that there are considerable variations in the treatment of the same illness by different doctors and in different areas. Since most patients are given the necessary treatment, though they may be on a waiting list for some time, these variations must – I believe – more often than not reflect overtreatment rather than undertreatment.

What do patients and the public at large think of such variations in medical practice? Not much, would be my view. Indeed, I would suggest that, in general, they are simply not aware of them. That situation will, I am sure, change in the future. The media will become more informed. We will see the formation of concerned patient groups. And to the extent that they argue against inappropriate and unnecessary treatment, they will certainly gain the attention of health insurance companies and of politicians wary of the burden on citizens of high taxes. Variations in medical practice will become an issue in public debate, at least as regards the more common procedures such as hysterectomy, prostatectomy, tonsillectomy, caesarean sections, etc., details of which are fairly easy to register and to process statistically.

The Western world is witnessing an increasing proportion of very well-educated people who are used to asking questions and bearing heavy responsibility in their working life. Many of them may also be influenced by the growth of an anti-authoritarian tradition in the last 20 years. They will not take the opinions of medical doctors as given, just because they wear the white vestiges of medical authority. They will know enough to ask the right questions and will sometimes even know the various answers. They will ask why they should have a particular treatment, especially if the cousin of their neighbour avoided such an operation for the (apparently) same diagnosis.

The public debate we had in Denmark in the summer of 1988 is symptomatic of what is to come. By chance, I think, it became known to the general public that some of the leading hospitals had randomised the treatment of breast cancer for research purposes over several years. Without being told about the randomisation, some women had the whole breast removed; others just the tumour. There was a public outcry. Why had the women not been told about the randomisation?

Another example is the intense public debate raging in Denmark at the time of writing (the spring of 1989). Should the Danish Parliament change the law and accept a new death criterion, based on brain rather than heart activity? The public seems not to accept that the recommendation to Parliament on this issue be given by doctors and other 'experts' alone.

In the same way, patients and the public will be increasingly concerned in future about medical treatment, including variations in the treatment of illnesses which are easy to monitor. Why should patients undergo a treatment which is unnecessary? Furthermore, even in circumstances where a particular treatment might be termed necessary, it may still be inappropriate, taking into consideration the total situation of a specific patient. For a 70-year-old an operation, or, perhaps more important, the postoperative effects, can be so risky that there may be a very real choice between the length of his or her remaining life and the better quality of a shorter life.

There is also the question of 'opportunity costs', as economists put it. Unnecessary treatment of one person may well lead to another person's having to wait for his necessary treatment. The resources of the health sector are not unlimited. Thus, unnecessary or inappropriate treatment of one person may harm not only this person, but also others. Unnecessary treatment is a waste of resources.

It follows that in future, doctors will have to be more open than they have been in the past about the treatment they propose. Is it necessary? Are there other treatment options? They will have to guide and inform the patient of what is best for him or her. The doctors will no longer have the sovereign right to decide what is best, but will have to consult the patients. In many cases the patient will have to be given a choice. Does he or she want an operation which may relieve him or her of symptoms, but which may be rather risky in itself, or which could have unpleasant side-effects?

For my part I never really thought about the existence of big variations in medical practice until I encountered the issue personally a few years ago. I knew about cases where the doctors were unable to diagnose an illness and therefore tried various treatments. I also knew about medical treatments substituting for traditional surgery, as with ulcers in the last couple of decades, both being supplied in the health market in parallel for some time. However, with a diagnosis to hand, I never thought two different hospitals would suggest two very different forms of treatment

As it happened, my mother became ill with myastenia gravis at the age of 74. It started with one of her eye-lids hanging down over the eye-apple. Luckily the eye specialist was knowledgeable enough to suggest a diagnosis of myastenia gravis – I have since read about patients going through a very trying time until the doctors are able to diagnose the illness – and referred her to a specialist, who was chief physician at the local (major) hospital. The specialist confirmed the diagnosis. It turned out that he had a special interest in this illness, having, as he told my mother, written an article in a medical journal on the treatment of myastenia gravis.

My mother was both physically and mentally in good shape. The chief physician told her that he would start with medical treatment but suggested that she should have an operation and the thymus removed. He did not say that the operation was absolutely necessary, but his advice was to have it done. As he later told me: 'If it were my own mother, I would advise her to have the operation.'

Luckily there is in Denmark a patients' association for myastenia gravis and a related group of muscle-nerve diseases. The hospital had given my mother an information sheet on the illness from this association. I called the secretariat of the association to ask for more information on the illness and its potential development. They referred me to their medical consultant, who happened to be a specialist at the National University Hospital in Copenhagen. I told him of my mother's diagnosis and asked him about the treatment. Initially I did not tell him that the specialist at her own hospital wanted her to be operated on, fearing that he might not feel free to give his own opinion.

The National University Hospital treats patients from about 60% of Denmark's 5 million population with this illness but not – normally – patients from my mother's region. The medical consultant to the patients' association said that the National Hospital would not normally operate on anybody with this illness over 50 years of age. His opinion was that the efficacy of the operation was uncertain. If effective, however, the full benefit might not be obtained for several years. Further, the medical treatment was promising. It would probably give my mother a good quality of life for her remaining years. The operation, on the other hand, was not a minor one and not without risk at her age.

My brother and I talked the matter over with our mother and suggested that she should not be operated on. We told her chief physician that we did not want the operation – without, of course, telling him we had also conferred with the consultant of the patients' association. He was annoyed and continued to press my mother to undergo the operation.

He continued medical treatment, however, and my mother's condition improved very noticeably. After some months the initial medical treatment started to lose its effect. She was hospitalised again. The doctor again suggested to my mother that she should be operated on. We refused again and he then started supplementing the initial treatment with cortisone. After a couple of weeks her condition was again much better. Thereafter the level of cortisone treatment was reduced. Then after a few weeks my mother's troubles started again because the reduction had gone too far. After that he sent her to the National Hospital for specific medication. My feeling was that he deliberately did not want the medical treatment to be a success. I may be wrong, of course.

I never understood, however, why the chief physician wanted to operate on my mother when he himself admitted at the time of the diagnosis that it was not a necessary treatment. Our suspicion was that he wanted her to be a case in his medical research.

When my mother was hospitalised, she met a 75-year-old man with the same illness, whom the doctor had operated on. If my brother and I had not intervened, my mother would certainly have been operated on too. It was difficult at her age and in her situation to oppose the wishes of the doctor.

I have given a rather detailed story of the treatment of my mother's illness because it illustrates several points.

What were the implications of telling my mother in the first place that an operation was not necessary, even though the doctor recommended it? Perhaps next time the doctor may feel he should just tell his patient that the operation is necessary. He may prefer not to involve his patient in the decision-making process. He had certainly not expected to be contradicted in the case of my mother.

What were the implications, then, for my mother? The refusal to be operated on caused her some problems, because the doctor continued to press her to undergo the operation. After all, might it not be effective in alleviating her illness? It was not an easy situation for her. And the chief physician certainly did not make it any easier because he did not respect our decision.

I was, luckily, in no doubt that our decision was right. But I could well imagine a situation where the relatives of a patient could, in such a situation, be in grave doubt about the choice between two treatments. What caused me some anger was that I dared not tell the chief physician as firmly as I wanted to that he should stop suggesting to my mother that she should be operated on.

The basic problem with practice variations seems to be the same as with health care in general: the suppliers of health care, i.e. the doctors, also play a central role in determining the level and type of treatment. The individual patient can not know what is good for him and cannot rationally select his own treatment. 'Supply side' responses, as economists would say, determine the treatment.

I think it would be helpful if some sort of medical ombudsman were established, one institution or more covering different illnesses, where patients could call for advice on treatment of a diagnosed illness. That would necessitate a group of doctors who would, if necessary, be prepared to contradict the verdict of their colleagues in the health care system.

Until it becomes a public issue, most people will probably not notice that there are various levels of treatment for the same illness. If they knew, they might well lose their trust in doctors and that would not necessarily be a good thing.

Certainly the issues involved here are important for patients and their families (as I have indicated in the case of my mother and our family), but they are just as important for the medical profession. We *want* to trust our doctors. But as more lay people like myself learn about medical practice variations, that trust is partly undermined. Unless doctors themselves act and are seen to act, then that trust will be undermined further. And that is in no one's interests.

CHAPTER 9

On the Need for Outcomes Research and the Prospects for the Evaluative Clinical Sciences

John E. Wennberg

INTRODUCTION

The extraordinary advances in the biomedical sciences are a proud accomplishment of our era, perhaps its most distinguished intellectual achievement. Yet, ironically, these advances in basic knowledge have increased uncertainty and intellectual confusion at the level that matters most to patients and physicians: clinical decisions concerning the treatments that are best for patients. The expansion of understanding of the nature of human biology and the mechanism of disease and the associated growth of a spectacular technology for intervening in biological processes has fostered the rapid proliferation of treatment theories on how to improve patient well-being. But, in contrast to the well-established public policies and administrative mechanisms for promoting growth of the biomedical sciences, support for the evaluative clinical sciences – the measurement sciences whose job it is to test the validity of clinical theories concerning the prevention, diagnosis and treatment of disease – has been inconsistent and unsystematic. The result of this neglect is clinical uncertainty concerning the expected outcomes of care and the value of care for patients.

THE DOUBLE STANDARD OF TRUTH

With the exception of the evaluation of new drugs, there is no mechanism in place to assure that major clinical theories are systematically evaluated. The nature of innovation in the pharmaceutical industry (where research proceeds in a reasonably orderly fashion from the bench to human experimentation) lends itself to regulatory approaches to establishing the effects drugs have on outcomes. The tightening of the regulatory process following the thalidomide and other drug-related therapeutic misadventures in 1960s led to a massive investment by the drug industry in the evaluation of new drugs, an investment that in most countries is recovered from patient dollars through the price of drugs. By contrast, the investigation of efficacy for other treatments where regulatory requirements have not been imposed is unsystematic; that which is undertaken results largely because someone is interested in the topic. Most of the funding comes through foundations or investigator-initiated grants financed from general revenue tax dollars.

The imbalance in emphasis on drug evaluation compared with all other treatment modalities can be measured by amounts of money allocated to assessments. About 1.5 billion dollars were spent in the USA in 1987 for drug trials, while the outcome research programme of the National Center for Health Services Research and Health Care Technology Assessment – the only formal assessment programme in the USA devoted to evaluation of all treatment theories relevant to a particular clinical condition – received an appropriation of only 6 million dollars in 1989.

The immediate consequence of the lack of attention to outcome assessment is an increasingly inadequate scientific basis for clinical decision making. The basic probabilities for the outcomes of specific treatments are often unknown or in controversy, and patients and physicians face unnecessary uncertainty in choosing among alternative treatments.

Let me give but three examples:

(1) The last few years have seen the rapid proliferation of medical theories concerning the best way to treat chest pain caused by impeded blood flow in the artery that feeds the muscle of the heart. Some physicians recommend surgery – the well-known coronary bypass operation. Others recommend coronary artery angioplasty – the insertion of a balloon catheter into the heart's artery which is then expanded to reduce the obstruction. Still others recommend drug treatment. Debates about the relative value of these different treatments rage in clinical medicine, but because the outcomes are not systematically compared, the debates cannot be settled.

(2) There are new ways to treat arthritis of the hip and knee. One approach involves the surgical replacement of the hip or knee joint, and for physicians and patients who choose this method there are a number of alternative ways of accomplishing the replacement. There are many choices but no consensus on which approach is best for the patient.

There is also considerable disagreement about when in the natural history of the disease the operation should be planned, if at all. These differences in opinion translate into costly differences in the rates at which various services are performed in different parts of the country.

(3) The evaluation of the outcomes of clinically different approaches to treating common medical conditions such as back pain, pneumonia and gastrointestinal disease is perhaps the most neglected area of all. In many communities physicians favour the outpatient setting for treating these patients, while in other communities the standards of practice favour the use of hospitals. Similar uncertainties and controversies about correct practice exist concerning the value of intensive care units.

CONSEQUENCES OF THE DOUBLE STANDARD

Neglect of these and a host of similar controversies about the scientifically and ethically correct way to practise medicine has enormous consequences for patient well-being and for the health care economy. Unresolved discrepancies in medical theory are responsible for much of the practice-style-driven influences on demand that affect the cost of use of care, even in medically sophisticated communities. Consider Boston and New Haven, which are internationally renowned centres of academic excellence in medicine. The residents of these two communities are remarkably similar in demographic characteristics that predict the need for care. They receive virtually all of their medical care from physicians affiliated with some of the world's finest medical schools. By definition, the medicine in these communities must be viewed as state of the art. But how different is the state of the art of medical thinking in these two communities, viewed from the perspective of what happens to patients:

> Residents of New Haven are about twice as likely to undergo a bypass operation for coronary artery disease as their counterparts in Boston, who are more likely to be treated by other means. On the other hand, Bostonians are·much more likely to have their hips and knees replaced by a surgical prosthesis than are New Havenites, whose physicians tend to prescribe medical treatment for these conditions. Bostonians are more than twice as likely to have a carotid endarterectomy – the controversial operation undertaken on the theory that it is the best way to prevent strokes arising from disease of the artery in the neck – while clinicians in New Haven appear to prefer medical management involving the daily use of aspirin or other drug. By contrast, hysterectomies for non-cancerous conditions of the uterus are more commonly performed on New Havenites.
>
> Most significant for the costs of medical care, Bostonians are much more likely to be hospitalised for medical conditions than are their counterparts

who live in New Haven. In 1982 Medicare reimbursements for hospitals were $1894 in Boston per person, while in New Haven they were $1078. If New Haven reimbursements had applied to the 78 000 enrollees living in Boston, the outlays would have been $63 million less – $85 million rather than the actual $148 million. Decisions on the best place to treat a host of acute and chronic medical conditions – the most common and costly examples of the differences are the treatment of low back pain, pneumonia and gastroenteritis – account for much of the differences in total per capita costs for medical care between these two communities. (Wennberg *et al.*, 1987.)

These statistics of variation carry broad implications. For many common conditions, the academic standards for medical practice as now constituted are not based on well-tested medical theory. Physicians, patients, those who pay for care and those in policy positions remain ignorant of the health care outcome consequences of spending vastly different proportions of the gross national product (GNP) on health care. The Boston–New Haven comparison shows that the scientific basis of medicine as now constituted does not distinguish the outcome significance of an investment of upwards of 16% of GNP (as for Bostonians) from 9% (as for New Havenites). Studies of practice variation in the international setting show that these North American patterns are the rule, not the exception. Similarly striking variations exist in rates of use of surgery among counties in Denmark and Norway, among cantons in Switzerland, among health districts in England and Scotland, to mention but a few of the increasing numbers of published reports of practice variations (Copenhagen Collaboration Center, 1985).

THE PROMISE OF THE EVALUATIVE CLINICAL SCIENCES

The statistics of variation are evidence of a deepening intellectual crisis in western medicine. Science, Thomas Kuhn argues, does not exist as a progressive, unified body of theory, knowledge and technique (Kuhn, 1970). Rather, there are multiple sciences, each making its appearance at times of intellectual crisis as a 'small' revolution, as a shift in 'paradigm' which establishes new disciplines in response to anomalies in theory or experimental evidence. A shift in paradigm involves new ways of posing problems and, often, new methods and techniques to address these problems; it requires exemplary research that provides models for how the disciplines should take their place as part of regular science.

Medicine is now experiencing such a Kuhnian revolution. Long-held assumptions about the efficacy, the ethical sufficiency and the legal basis of the physician's role in making vicarious utility assessments for patients, as well as the validity of many specific theories physicians hold on appropriate practice, are now recognised as problematic. Professional uncertainty rather than consensus about the scientific basis of clinical practice is emerging as the dominating reality (Wennberg *et al.*, 1982). More and more, patients are demanding to participate as active partners in the decisions that determine their medical fates. At the same time, new methods and technologies and exemplary applications of these techniques to problems of professional uncertainty also are emerging. It is now possible to speak about a new set of disciplines that together constitute the evaluative clinical sciences. They offer the promise of a scientific programme that can greatly decrease uncertainty about the probabilities and the value to patients of the outcomes of care, and can improve the information base for clinical as well as policy decisions.

A number of important disciplinary advances contribute to the evaluative sciences.

First, advances in statistical theory and methods make it possible to manage new classes of problems relevant to predicting outcomes and testing theories about alternative treatments. These advances, which permit statistical adjustments for differences in severity of illness in the study of outcomes, are useful for measuring the quality of care and for assessing outcomes in non-experimental study designs.

Second, advances in medical care epidemiology make it possible to use health insurance claims data and other large data systems to monitor the use and outcome of care in specific locations and to base postgraduate education and quality assurance programmes on the feedback of measures of performance. Claims data technology also provides new methods for estimating outcome probabilities with improved accuracy and at lowered costs. The claims data systems also represent a registry of medical care events and can be used to locate patients efficiently for follow-up studies, thus offering additional ways of lowering the cost of outcome studies.

Third, advances in psychometrics have provided standardised valid measure of patient symptoms and functional status ('quality of life'), opening up new domains for assessing outcomes. These developments are particularly significant for evaluating surgical theory when the reasons for surgery are to improve the quality of life.

Fourth, decision analysis, adapted to medical decision making and applied to a series of prototypical clinical decision problems, allows objective testing of clinical theories through simulated experimentations. It also provides a means for assessing the importance of uncertainties about the true probabilities for specific outcomes and for evaluating the importance of patient utilities in a specific clinical choice.

Fifth, advances in information technology have enormous significance for the evaluative sciences. It is now possible, using the personal computer, to make calculations and conduct analyses that 10 years ago were only possible on large, expensive mainframe computers. Physicians in their offices and on the wards of hospitals can now have at their fingertips the computing power necessary to obtain 'real time', precise and specific information relevant to the medical care decisions of their individual patients.

Finally, progress in the related area of interactive, computer-driven video disc technology and conceptual breakthroughs in accessing and presenting information provides revolutionary new ways for synthesising, conveying and individualising information that can support a luxurious and active cross-communication between the patient and the physician. Through video and other graphic means, patients can see vignettes of the possible futures they face, according to the treatments they may choose. Thus, the technology holds the promise of activating the patient as a partner in the decision process. This will be particularly useful when the choice involves complex trade-offs that require evaluation of patient preferences or utilities, such as the decision to live with symptoms or to undergo a risky treatment in the expectation of reducing symptoms.

AN EXAMPLE OF OUTCOMES RESEARCH

Let me give a concrete example of how the evaluative clinical sciences can be used to evaluate medical theory and activate patient participation in the decision process. At issue is the treatment of prostatism or obstruction of the urinary tract due to benign hypertrophy of the prostate gland or BPH.* BPH is a very common condition, affecting the majority of men by the time they reach the seventh or eight decade of life.

One common treatment for BPH is an operation, a prostatectomy. The use of prostatectomy shows striking variations among neighbouring communities, so that in some places about 10% of men undergo this operation by age 85, while in other communities the proportion can be as high as 50%. The treatment is the most expensive major operation paid for by Medicare – the federal insurance programme in the USA for patients 65 years of age and older. Programme outlays for hospitalisation costs and surgery fees in 1985 were well over a billion dollars.

Another common treatment for BPH is watchful waiting. In communities with low rates of prostatectomy, proportionately more men

*Reports of the assessment were published in May of last year as a four-part series in the *Journal of the American Medical Association*, **259**(20), 27 May 1988.

with BPH are treated by this alternative strategy, which emphasises the viewpoint that prostatectomy is an elective procedure, reserved for those with truly bothersome symptoms.

Four years ago our research and physicians participating in Maine's Medical Assessment program formed an assessment team to consider the causes of variations in rates of prostatectomy among Maine communities. These discussions (and a review of the scientific papers published on BPH) uncovered an important and unsettled controversy concerning the indications for the operation:

Many physicians hold to the theory that prostatectomy should be performed early in the course of BPH as a preventive measure. They reason that if the operation is delayed, the patient will be older and be at higher risk when the operation finally becomes unavoidable; if the operation is delayed, life expectancy is reduced. For most patients, according to this theory, watchful waiting is not a reasonable option.

Other physicians argue that the need for the operation is not inevitable, that for most patients it does not improve life expectancy and that the primary reason for an operation for such patients is the relief of symptoms and improvement in the quality of life. According to this theory, watchful waiting is a reasonable option for patients who prefer to live with their symptoms in order to avoid the risk of the operation.

The assessment team tested this conflict in theory, to reach several conclusions. Using evidence from the literature and from claims data, the assessment demonstrated that the preventive theory was wrong: an operation in patients with uncomplicated BPH – and most patients are like this – very likely causes a slight decrease in life expectancy. Thus, the assessment confirmed the opinion of those physicians who felt that the operation was justified on the basis of its value for reducing symptoms and improving the qualtity of life. Interview studies with patients before and at 3, 6 and 12 months after surgery documented symptom and functional status changes in relation to the operation and showed that the value of the operation for most patients rests in its superior effect over watchful waiting in reducing symptoms and improving the quality of life. But these gains are available only to patients willing to take the risks of the operation, which include death, failure to improve symptoms, impotence and incontinence. Thus, the decision to undergo the operation is highly dependent on patients' preferences for outcomes and attitudes towards risk.

By clarifying controversies, establishing correct theory and providing detailed probability estimates for the full spectrum of relevant outcomes, some of which had not been previously studied, the assessment has immediate practical value for improving clinical decision making. The practice-style-related causes of variation in prostatectomy rates were traced to an incorrect belief in the preventive theory of early pros- tatectomy and failure to take patient preferences into account in recommending prostatectomy. The remedy for unwanted practice style variations, we concluded, required the active engagement of the patient in the decision. It involves informing physicians and patients of the risks and benefits of prostatectomy and its alternative, watchful waiting.

We are testing the value of interactive video-disc technology as a remedy for unwanted, practice style variations. Our prototype 'Pros- tatectomy Shared Patient Decision-making Procedure' has three goals:

(1) Meet the legal and ethical requirements for information that are scientifically accurate, emotively balanced and fair to the different treatment alternatives.

(2) Improve the scientific basis of medicine by providing a method for continuously updating the estimates of the outcome probabilities used to inform patients.

(3) Provide the research framework for learning how to help patients understand their choices and make better decisions.

The interactive computer-driven audiovisual disc is designed to be administered in the physician's office with little or no assistance from medical personnel other than an initial data entry phase of standardised information on health status and physical condition. The patient is also asked to answer questions about the symptoms, his functional status and the strength of his feelings about them. These data are used in two ways: (1) to identify the relevant prognostic subgroup to which the patient belongs, so that the information presented to him is the best available estimate; and (2) to enroll the patient in the prospective study of outcomes.

The patient is then presented with an audiovisual narration depicting the choices he faces, their various possible outcomes and associated probabilities. Interviews with two physician-patients (one who chose watchful waiting and the other prostatectomy) convey to the patient that he indeed has a choice: if physicians choose differently, so can their patients. Other interviews are testimonies about the principal outcomes, including an example of a complication associated with either choice. The interactive computer feature of the Shared Decision-making Proce- dure means that information on the probabilities for outcomes pre- sented to the patient are specific to his subgroup, according to symptom severity and age. The patient can also exercise options to learn more about issues of particular concern as well as review what he has seen. At the end, he is given a printed synopsis of what he has seen, to discuss with his family and physician. The physician then helps the patient to make his decision.

The patient returns later (e.g. after 3, 6 or 24 months), regardless of type of treatment, when additional information about his health and satisfaction with his choice is obtained and entered into the database. These data, accumulated over time and for many patients, are then used by researchers to update the information presented to the patient. In this way, the expert system participates in its own update and helps improve the scientific basis of medicine. Protocols are also planned to help patients to understand better their own preferences and excercise them in the decision process.

PRINCIPLES TO GUIDE THE MANDATE TO EXTEND SYSTEMATIC ASSESSMENTS

The need is for a broad extension of the mandate to evaluate medical interventions to include the full spectrum of relevant treatments, clinical theories and outcomes. The mandate must expand to include diagnostic and therapeutic procedures and established drugs used in novel ways, as well as the use of hospitals and intensive care units compared with their alternatives. In addition to traditional measures of mortality, morbidity and physiological or biochemical parameters of outcome, good outcomes research requires good measures of symptoms and how treatment affects them. It also depends on functional status and quality of life measures, outcome measures that are increasingly important as, more and more, the stated objectives of many medical interventions are the reduction of symptoms and improvement in well-being.

Extending the mandate to evaluate the outcomes of all relevant treatment options presents a challenge to the research and practice communities, funding agencies and policy makers. The nature of the assessment problems and the way innovation occurs in most fields of medicine suggest certain principles to guide this effort.

(1)   Assessments Must Be Conducted According to the Principles of 'Regular Science' As Part of Systems of Organised, Peer-reviewed Medical Research

The uncertainties we are talking about are fundamentally scientific uncertainties which can only be resolved by obtaining information and using it to test theories. The needed improvements in the scientific basis of clinical decision making depend on these assessments, and they must proceed in an orderly fashion to develop a body of knowledge based on proven rules of evidence and formally structured peer review. Outcome assessments are not 'demonstration' projects. The intellectual rigour now commonplace in the biomedical sciences must be the standard. In the final analysis, the authority and effectiveness of the assessments depend solely on their credibility as objective science. The principle of scientific independence is essential as the protection that assures a balanced, unbiased source of information about what is known and what remains controversial in the evolution of clinical theory. It will be difficult, if not impossible, to obtain this independence if the agency responsible for sponsoring outcome assessments has an active role in the management of health care systems or represents some faction in the competition for truth.

(2) Assessments Must Be Ongoing: the Nature of Innovation in Medicine Requires Continuous Evaluation and Re-evaluation As New Theories Arise

Innovation in medicine is dynamic and the need for assessments is an iterative, ongoing one. Information needs continuous updating and improvement; (new assessments will be needed as new theories develop and old ones evolve. The BPH assessment team uncovered several new treatment theories which need assessment. We found a new approach to BPH based on the use of microwaves to shrink the prostate; a new, less invasive, operative approach based on a simple incision of the gland; and a new idea that BPH can be treated with a balloon that is expanded to push the prostate tissue aside (an adaptation of angioplasty technology). We also learned about drugs which may work. These theories need testing. Our experience suggests the need for assessment teams to have ongoing responsibility to keep abreast of new developments and to perform (or influence others to perform) adequate studies. Their recommendation on the need for randomised clinical trials offers further guidance to the rational evaluation of medical theory. Like their counterparts in biomedical research, the scientists involved need to make career investments in a problem area. The experience and knowledge are accumulative. Assessment projects dealing with major human illness such as BPH need to be continued indefinitely.

(3) Priorities Must Be Set: the Assessments Done First Must Be Those That Matter Most

The assessment projects that are established first should be those that matter most to patients and to those who are concerned with the quality of care and the allocation of scarce resources. Most would agree that the

Table 9.1   Suggested priority conditions or illnesses for patient outcome research program

Condition	Treatment controversies
Stable angina	Bypass surgery vs angioplasty vs drugs
Unstable angina	Bypass surgery vs angioplasty vs drugs
Arteriosclerosis causing stroke	Endarterectomy vs drugs
Peripheral vascular disease	Bypass surgery vs angioplasty vs medical management
Lens extraction	(by type of surgery) vs watchful waiting
Gallstones	Surgery vs stone crushing vs medical management vs watchful waiting
Arthritis of the hip and knee	Surgery (by type) vs medical management
Non-cancerous conditions of the uterus	Surgery (by type) vs hormone treatment vs watchful waiting
Prostatism	Surgery (by type) vs angioplasty vs drugs vs watchful waiting
Ear, nose and throat conditions	Surgery (by type) vs various drugs
Herniated disc	Surgery vs various medical treatments
Acute and chronic medical conditions:	
Back pain/strain	Hospitalisation vs ambulatory-based care; ICU vs usual ward care
Gastroenteritis	
Respiratory disease	
Heart disease	

focus needs to be on testing the alternative ways of dealing with common medical problems for which at least one treatment option is knows to be costly and/or risky. The nominations in Table 9.1 are reasonable. Even though the list of priority illnesses or conditions is small, it covers the large majority of costly variations in surgery and hospitalisation, such as those illustrated by the New Haven–Boston comparisons. Assessments in these areas would affect most patients who are now, according to some theories, candidate for surgery or hospitalisation.

(4)   Regulation Will Not Work: Innovation for Most Medical Treatments is Decentralised and Assessments Not Easily Mandated through Formal Regulation

The mandate to extend evaluations to the use of surgery, diagnostic tests and hospitals cannot be accomplished through regulation. There is an essential difference between the research and development strategies of the drug industry and the dynamics of innovation for most medical practices. Drugs follow a linear process of technology development and assessment, from the bench to the animal laboratory and, finally, to human experimentation. The mandate to evaluate is easily accomplished through regulation tied to the licence to market and the resources needed for evaluation are provided as part of corporate policy. But most medical innovations develop as part of the problem-solving activity of physicians in their daily encounters with patients, in decentralised environments where there are few resources available for evaluation. The uses now made of hospitals and intensive care units, as well as many surgical operations, are good examples. It would not be easy to subject such practice conventions to formal regulation, simply because there is no clear distinction between 'regular' practice and innovation. Moreover, because the innovators often are individuals or members of small groups and their products are not generally patentable, they have little capital and little incentive to invest their own resources in outcomes evaluation. The result of a serious effort to regulate innovation would almost certainly be the stifling of innovation.

Assessment teams are suggested as an alternative to regulation in a situation where regulation is not likely to succeed. They accomplish their mandate for evaluation because team members are drawn to the intellectual, scientific and ethical questions of efficacy and because their professional careers are vested in the evaluative clinical sciences.

(5) Stable Funding Must Be Assured

Unlike biomedical science, which has been amply funded from general tax revenues, support for the clinical evaluative sciences has been inconsistent and eclectic. In North America the charitable foundations have played a major role, but the interest of foundations is in demonstration projects, not in sustaining a research programme that serves a vital and on-going societal need. The exception to the lack of stable programme money, as mentioned above, is the funds available for new drug assessments. These monies, recovered through the price of drugs, in effect represent a tax on patient care dollars and can be viewed as an investment in further development of the products that matter most to patients – the treatments they receive. An extension of this tax to pay for evaluation of all treatment theories is a fair and reasonably easy way to raise the necessary investments. In the USA the amount of the tax on patient care dollars needed to sustain an active programme in outcomes research has been estimated at between 0.1 and 0.2% of medical care expenditures (*c.* 200–400 million US dollars per annum).

(6) Rapid Completion Is Essential: Assessments Must Produce Useful Results Within Reasonable Time

The principle 'quick is beautiful' I borrow from Freeman Dyson (Dyson, 1988), who notes that projects that are timely and offer results in a few years succeed, while those with longer time-frames tend to fail. The notion of the assessment team fits this principle well. The utility of the assessment team's studies does not depend on large-scale randomised clinical trials. As the prostatectomy assessment illustrates, substantial clarification of clinical theory is possible on the basis of non-experimental studies alone.

PROSPECTS

The failure of the investigator-initiated grant mechanism to meet the challenge of outcome assessment has led to a programme in the USA that embodies these principles and provides one model of how a research programme might be built. The outcomes research programme of the National Center for Health Services Research and Health Care Technology Assessment, beginning in 1989, will fund assessment teams that accept responsibility for evaluating alternative treatment theories for specific common disease conditions such as prostatism or stable angina. The interdisciplinary teams, composed of clinical investigators, epidemiologists, practising physicians and others with relevant skills in the evaluative clinical sciences, are required by the terms of their grant awards to keep track of treatment innovations in their area of responsibility and undertake for all treatments the equivalent of phase I and phase II assessments now required for drugs. On the basis of their assessments, the teams are to identify priority clinical trials (phase III studies) that are needed. Their conclusions and recommendations will be published on a periodic basis. They are also responsible for conducting phase IV studies.* Funding for the programme is from patient

---

*The language is adapted from that used in the assessment of new drugs: phase I studies are primarily designed to demonstrate the safety of an intervention; phase II studies are to obtain indicative evidence for effectiveness, sufficient to establish the ethical and scientific necessity for further study; Phase III are 'definitive' tests of efficiency (i.e. those which in the case of new drugs provide the evidence needed for approval for marketing – usually, large-scale prospective clinical trials). Phase IV studies are surveillance studies done after marketing. While phase I and II studies have not been systematically done for most treatments now in common use, the assessment teams will find considerably more information available for evaluation than is the case for new drugs. The prostatism assessment described above illustrates how the existing literature, claims data, functional status measures and decision analysis can be used to conduct (using a non-experimental approach) the equivalent of a phase II study. (Wennberg *et al.*, 1988.)

dollars – from the Medicare trust fund. Priorities are according to common conditions, for which at least one current treatment arm poses particularly high costs and/or risks for Medicare enrollees. About 15 teams will be needed to cover the majority of surgery and medical hospitalisations.

The programme provides a non-regulatory model for assuring that systematic outcome assessments are accomplished. How the information on outcome is used will depend on other mechanisms, agencies or incentives. The goal of outcomes research is better clinical science – to establish the facts and test theory – not to make specific regulatory determinations. The assessments of health care outcomes conducted under the programme will challenge the theories and practice patterns of the nation's physicians, but the challenge will be on the high ground of scientific evidence and an imperative all physicians recognise – the need to do what is best for patients.

What about the prospects for the evaluative clinical sciences in outcomes research in medical schools? The reformers of the Flexnarian* period, successful in so many dimensions in their quest to improve the scientific basis of medicine, failed to identify a clear role for the evaluative sciences. In many medical schools the curriculum is virtually devoid of formal exposure to critical thinking about the logical and evidentiary requirements for inference in clinical medicine. Training in clinical epidemiology, decision analysis, computer science and the measurement of health care outcomes is characteristically undervalued. While postgraduate training for clinicians in these disciplines has been successfully fostered by the charitable foundations (such as the clinical scholars programme), the teachers are characteristically members of the faculty of schools of public health, not medical schools. However, the situation is now changing. Consistent with Kuhn's model for normalisation of science, there is a struggle to define the role and mode of presence of the evaluative clinical sciences with the formal structures and relationships of the medical schools and academic medical centres. The evaluative clinical sciences are beginning to be nurtured and taught in the medical schools. New experiments in curricula are under way notably at McMaster University and now Harvard University. New departments or centres for the evaluative clinical sciences are developing – for example, at Harvard and Dartmouth. These developments can be read as signs for the improved prospect of the evaluative clinical sciences as part of 'regular' medical science.

There is a need for international collaboration in the development of the clinical evaluative sciences and the agenda for outcomes research.

---

* Abraham Flexner, a non-medical researcher, critic and writer, brought about major reforms in the quality of modern medical and science education in the United States.

The hallmark of the current situation is a localised, particularistic approach to the development of clinical science, a situation that contrasts strikingly with the international community of scientists that constitutes the biomedical sciences. The established exception, again, is in the field of drug evaluation, where several important co-operative international trials have been undertaken.

Over the past 3 years, the Copenhagen Collaboration Center (CCC) has amply demonstrated the advantages of an international approach to the assessment team concept discussed above. The CCC organised researchers from the UK, Scandinavia, Holland, Israel, Canada and the USA to develop protocols and pool data from national or regional registries or from claims data for assessments of prostatectomy, cholecystectomy and hysterectomy. Treatment theories related to the use of these operations vary substantially from physician to physician within a country, but even more so between countries, and the CCC has been able to take advantage of this wider range of practice patterns in its assessments. Prostatectomy again provides a good example.

A prostatectomy can be accomplished as an 'open' operation requiring an incision of the skin and the complete removal of the obstructing prostate tissue, or as a 'TURP' (Transurethral Resection of the Prostate), using a resectoscope introduced through the urethra. The TURP has replaced the open prostatectomy as the treatment favoured by most physicians in the USA and most of Europe, but in certain parts of Canada and Israel the open operation remains popular. This shift in surgical theory and practice occurred without formal assessment of the outcomes of these two ways of treating prostatism. But the CCC research group found that registry or claims data were available over the lifetime of the shift in technology and, using claims and registry data, were able to make comparisons of the outcomes of these two approaches to prostatectomy at different time periods and among different countries. Analysis of these data shows that operative failure – measured by the need for a second prostatectomy, subsequent diagnostic examination and incidence of strictures – is substantially higher following TURP. The research raises the uncomfortable possibility that the more effective technology may have been replaced. The CCC team has recommended that a prospective trial of open prostatectomy versus TURP should be undertaken (in places where the open operation is still performed).

The expansion of outcomes research in Europe will require the identification of reliable sources of funds, methods for setting priorities and strategies for insuring the scientific integrity of evaluative research. As in North America, clinical epidemiology, decison analysis, computer sciences and other aspects of the evaluative clinical sciences need to be part of the basic education of the modern physician, and researchers, teachers and clinicians proficient in these skills must find rewarding careers in medical schools. The prospect for achieving these objectives as well as for international collaboration will be enhanced when academic medical centres in Europe move to establish departments or centres for the evaluative clinical sciences.

ACKNOWLEDGEMENTS

The work described in this chapter has been funded in part by The National Center of Health Services Research and the John A. Hartford Foundation. Parts of this chapter are adapted from an article which appeared in *Health Affairs* (Spring, 1988) and from congressional testimony given by the author before the Committee on Finance, Senate Finance Subcommittee on Health, 11 July 1988.

REFERENCES

CCC Bibliography on Regional Variations in Health Care (1985). Copenhagen Collaborating Center

Dyson, F. J. (1988). *Infinite in All Directions: An Explanation of Science and Belief.* Harper & Row, New York

Kuhn, T. (1970). *The Structure of Scientific Revolutions*, 2nd edn. University of Chicago Press, Chicago

Wennberg, J. E., Barnes, B. A. and Zubkoff, M. (1982). Professional uncertainty and the problem of supplier-induced demand. *Soc. Sci. Med.*, **16**, 811–24

Wennberg, J. E., Freeman, J. L. and Culp, W. J. (1987). Are hospital services rationed in New Haven or over-utilized in Boston? *Lancet*, 23 May, 1185, 1189

Wennberg, J. E., Mulley, A., Hanley, D. *et al.* (1988). As assessment of prostatectomy for benign urinary tract obstruction. *J. Am. Med. Ass.*, **259**(20), 3027–30

CHAPTER 10

Promoting Clinical Policy Change: Using the Art To Promote the Science in Medicine

Jonathan Lomas

> To the physician particularly a scientific discipline is an incalculable gift, which leavens his whole life, giving exactness to habits of thought and tempering the mind with that judicious faculty of distrust which can alone, amid the uncertainties of practice, make him wise unto salvation. For perdition inevitably awaits the mind of the practitioner ... who has never grasped clearly the relations of science to his art, and who knows nothing, and perhaps cares less, for the limitations of either.
>
> Sir William Osler, 1894

MEDICAL PRACTICE: THE SCIENTIFIC ART OR THE ARTISTIC SCIENCE?

At the time of Sir William Osler, the task at hand was to remind practitioners and public alike that medicine had a scientific basis at all. How the pendulum has swung. The years of the twentieth century have seen the public and profession become comfortable with, and indeed presume, the notion of medicine as science, and the task is now to remind all that medicine still has a significant component of 'art' (Greer, 1987). The phenomenal increase in the role of the basic sciences in medical research, the proliferation of exacting technologies, the ever-burgeoning knowledge base found in journals, and the messages given by the profession itself, all present a coherent image of medicine as an engineering concept in which symptom x is carefully diagnosed as caused by factor y, which will yield with assured probabilities to treatment z. There is no room for the art of medicine in the image, for if there were, there would be an acceptance of discretion, of fallibility, of uncertainty, and of apparent irrationality and inconsistency in the practice of medicine. With such acceptance would come questions of effectiveness of all that is done in the name of medicine, and of the advisability of public financial support for all that is contained within that Pandora's box of 'medical practice'.

In fact, the growing dismay over medical practice variations is sign and symbol of the pendulum's swing back to a recognition of the art in medicine, and thus a recognition of the limits of medicine (and, potentially, the limits of the public's funding of medicine). Herein lies the paradox for the medical profession. On the one hand, they see the dangers of letting the artist cat out of the medical science bag; on the other hand, they see both the reality and the power of individual discretion over each medical act. Without individual discretion (the 'art' of medicine) they become technocrats, not professionals; with individual discretion they produce the kind of variations at the aggregate level that is the subject of this book, and they lay themselves open to scepticism, reduced status and careful investigation of the contents of the Pandora's box by those from 'outside'.

The correct image of medical practice is obviously one of both art and science and, as Osler states, 'the limitations of either'. Medical practice variations are one indication of the extent to which it is still an art. Because we have tended to lose sight of (or have had obfuscated for us) the art in medicine, we are surprised and even shocked at medical practice variations. This loss of sight has also clouded the basis upon which we view medical policy. This is true for both public policy and clinical policy. In the public policy arena the rediscovery of significant discretion over the amount of resources required to achieve equivalent health outcomes – so aptly termed 'conservative' versus 'elaborate' practice styles by McClure (1982) – is very recent and is only now leading to economic incentives to leverage the art of medicine towards conservative practice styles. Diagnostic Related Groupings, decentralised physician budgeting, and the general thrust of 'managed care' are the beginnings of this new era.

In clinical policy the change in view is yet slower and the assumptions of science still predominate. Clinical policies form the backbone of medical practice (Eddy, 1982). When we observe practice variations, it is because the physicians of one community have adopted a different clinical policy for one set of indications compared with physicians of another community. But where do these clinical policies come from? How are they formed and how are they communicated? The common language of communication among physicians is the 'scientific literature', which exists at a supra national level in today's internationalised world of medicine. It is available (within reason) to the same extent and with the same message to all physicians, regardless of the community in which they practise. A prominent mode of thinking has been that publication in this literature of evidence on new procedures, new drugs or new therapies is absorbed quickly and appropriately into clinical practice. By this reasoning one should not expect to see variations in practice, because the same information is available to all as they construct their clinical policies.

This view of the physician as the rational information-seeking and implementing 'scientist' is, however, far from complete. The uncertainty around the applicability of results from a research study to a particular patient, the economic incentives of the system in which the physician operates, the views and practices of colleagues in the community, predilections traceable to the educational background of the physician, the administrative rules and regulations of the local and system-wide environment, and the knowledge and nature of the patient population the physician serves will all conspire often to make the clinical policy that is actually adopted only distantly related to what is indicated by the common pool of scientific research evidence in an area of practice (Lomas and Haynes, 1988).

Therefore, not only do clinical policies often bear only a slight resemblance to science, but also the extent and nature of their divergence from the evidence will vary according to the local characteristics of the community in which the physician practises. It is not that physicians fail to act as scientists at all – they are often aware of the research evidence – but rather that this is only one of the roles in which they see themselves. Colleague to their local peers, advocate for their patients, adherent to their hospital's rules, member of their profession (and specialty), and agent for their own economic interests are all competing roles with that of scientist. These are the competing roles that, when combined, make up the art of medicine. Eisenberg has noted that individual physicians' clinical policies are determined by 'a multiplicity of interacting factors, [and] that much of the variation in medical practice is due to physician's attempts to satisfy their personal desires and simultaneously to serve as their patients' agents' (Eisenberg, 1986: p. 79).

Thus, the *potential* for medical practice to be scientific has been sold as reality. The reality is medicine more as art than as science, and medical practice variations are announcing to the world that the emperor has no clothes. The most obvious implication of this announcement is that the mere publication of new knowledge in the scientific literature, or even drawing specific attention to this literature, will usually be inadequate in changing clinical policy (Lomas, 1988). We must better understand the relative impact of the scientific literature, the national and, most important, the local environment of medical practice if we are to promote changes in clinical policy which move it closer to a reflection of the scientific evidence. By adopting this approach we will have recognised that the balance of medical practice is not currently scientific, but that judicious use of the components of practice which are medical art can, paradoxically, promote appropriate clinical policy change.

In the next section the array of influences on clinical policies is described, with particular stress on the distinction between national (or distant) influences and local (or proximal) influences. This is followed by an analysis of how these influences can be exploited by the medical profession itself to promote more appropriate clinical policies; a case study of our own work is included for illustration. Finally, the likely alternative of government and third-party regulation of medical practice is outlined, and it is posited that lack of action by the medical profession would make this alternative inevitable.

THE INFLUENCES ON CLINICAL POLICY

In better understanding the influences on clinical policies – in order to evaluate how to change them – it is useful to know at least three characteristics of them. First, where does the influence come from? With the exception of scientific evidence itself, most influences emanate from either the national/regional environment which determines the overall structure of the health care system, or from the local community which determines the atmosphere of practice (Greer, 1988). Second, what is the route through which the influence occurs? Is it administrative systems, educational experiences, economic incentives or patients' predilections (Lomas and Haynes, 1988)? Finally, what is the impact of these influences on clinical policies? We can borrow from psychology to characterise this influence as predisposing, enabling or reinforcing change (Green and Eriksen, 1988).

There has been an accumulation of evidence in recent years on the influences on clinical policy, such that it is possible to list an impressive array of these contributions to the art of medicine. Table 10.1 outlines such a list according to the first two of the above variables – the route and the source of the influence. The evidence in support of these factors as contributors to clinical policy will not be reviewed in detail here, because it is available in a number of places elsewhere (for reviews see, for example, Eddy, 1982; Winkler *et al.*, 1985; Eisenberg, 1985, 1986; Schroeder, 1987; Lomas and Haynes, 1988). In general, they are best seen as an interacting set: no single influence (with the possible exception of economic incentives) has an overriding effect, but in combination they are powerful determinants of medical practice.

Under the heading of 'source of the influence' it should be noted that

Table 10.1 The source and route of influences on an individual physician's clinical policies

Route of influence	Source of influence	
	National	*Local*
Patients	Malpractice attitudes Health status of population	Level of knowledge Age–sex profile Socioeconomic status Health status of patients
Education	Scientific literature Official policies Medical training system Licensing requirements Media Commercial advertising Continuing medical education courses	Hospital rounds Educational influentials/ leaders Medical school where trained[a] Specialty training[a] Time since graduation[a] Pharmaceutical/other 'detailing' Colleagues' views
Administrative factors	Organisation and structure of health care system Claims monitoring systems Data-reporting requirements Drug formularies Activities of disciplinary bodies Explicit rationing rules Health-related legislation	Hospital policies Peer review/audit activities Practice setting, e.g. group/ solo Availability of technology Hospital medical staff organisation Performance data Hospital bed capacity
Economic	Remuneration system, e.g. fee-for-service/salary Relative values of fee items Inclusion/exclusion of fee items Prospective/retrospective reimbursement	Physician supply density

[a] These are not strictly characteristics of the local environment, but rather personal characteristics of the physician.

most of the national factors provide a background landscape upon which the details of the picture can be painted by the local community influences. For example, national media coverage of (say) cholesterol screening is unlikely to influence a physician's clinical policy unless there are local facilities to do such screening, colleagues are also adopting screening policies and/or local patients are requesting such screening. Similarly, national demonstration of practice variations will not influence clinical policy unless it is revealed at the level of the physician's community and in a context that is relevant to the physician's actual practice conditions (Wennberg *et al.*, 1977).

These observations are congruent with the thorough work of Greer, who has recently published the results of over 200 interviews with physicians from three countries aimed at uncovering the influences on their chosen practice patterns (Greer, 1988). Not only does she reiterate the conclusions of Eisenberg that there is a complex interaction of influences, but also she highlights the overriding importance of the local community in determining what is acceptable as a clinical policy. Community practitioners do not 'trust' information – research studies or otherwise – that is national in origin without local consensus and validation by their colleagues. Not surprisingly, it is the everyday experiences and the everyday contacts that are the most powerful influences on behaviour.

This should not be taken to mean that there is no influence from the national level factors. The early studies of surgical rate variations (e.g., Vayda, 1973) were comparisons of national level variations, with the implied causation of different payment systems because the higher rates were seen in the countries with the overservicing incentive of fee-for-service payment. More recently this national influence has been elegantly demonstrated in a study of the policies adopted for coronary artery bypass surgery and coronary angiography among expert panels of US versus UK physicians (Brook *et al.*, 1988). The UK physicians consistently set their threshold for surgical intervention higher than their US colleagues, indicating that their educational experience, the national level payment and/or administrative structure of the UK system had an overall 'dampening' effect on their propensity to resort to surgical intervention.

Nevertheless, these influences are the colour washes that suggest the landscape, not the fine brushwork of the detailed painting. The only way such influences appear to have a specific effect is when the economic or administrative incentives available through a national payment scheme can be targeted at a particular clinical practice. In the Canadian province of Quebec the alteration of the relative value of fee items through the fee schedule had a major impact on the use of home visits across the province (Barer *et al.*, 1988). In the UK, regional health authority administrative policies on eligibility criteria for procedures such as renal dialysis or hip replacement also have an impact on the use of these procedures.

The importance of the local as opposed to the national environment, except perhaps for direct economic and regulatory incentives, also comes through clearly when the effectiveness of different strategies for changing policy is analysed according to the route of influence. In most cases strategies have attempted to target only one of the routes of influence on practice, and these routes have tended to be identified with particular constituencies in the health care system. Internally the medical profession has relied almost entirely on the educational route, with publication of research and offerings of traditional continuing medical education as the predominant strategies. This is entirely congruent with the public image of the physician as 'scientist', acquiring information rationally and making probabilistic decisions. However, dissemination of research through traditional continuing medical education has now been shown to be largely ineffective in changing clinical behaviour (Haynes *et al.*, 1984; Schroeder *et al.*, 1984). Indeed, the mere provision of educational information does not change clinical policies, whether it is provided nationally through consensus conference reports (Kosecoff *et al.*, 1987; Hill *et al.*, 1988), or through guidelines for practice (Retchin *et al.*, 1985), or even through carefully designed and mailed packages (Avorn and Soumerai, 1983; Evans *et al.*, 1986). However, this information does appear to increase awareness of the appropriate policy, even if it is not acted upon (Jacoby and Clark, 1986; Kosecoff *et al.*, 1987).

Similar findings exist for hospitals which have relied almost entirely on the administrative route. Traditional medical audit, in which there are the implicit criteria of peer review, little or no feedback on performance at the local level and no corrective follow-up action, does not change behaviour.

To the extent that governments or third party payers have involved themselves at all in trying to have an impact on clinical policies, it has been primarily through the route of economic incentives. More on this later. Patient-centred strategies have been favoured by few, with the possible exception of health promotion areas of practice, where patient education is not so much directed at changing physicians' clinical policies as at changing patients' life-styles – an equally challenging task!

After reviewing this literature, it has become clear that most strategies have failed to appreciate the multiplicity of interacting influences on physicians' clinical policies, and therefore have failed to achieve any change in the policies. The few successful strategies have targeted an array of influences from both the educational and administrative routes. The optimal approaches appear to be ones that 'incorporate personalized education of practitioners by respected peers, coupled with structured feedback (computerised or not) on subsequent audited performance' (Lomas and Haynes, 1988: p. 1). Once again the importance of the local community in determining final clinical policies is highlighted.

It is now that the importance of categorising into predisposing, enabling and reinforcing influences emerges. Many of the traditional single-route approaches, often emanating from the national level, appear to predispose physicians towards change, but it is the local and personalised influences that actually enable and then reinforce changes in clinical policy. Thus, it is not that (say) continuing medical education has no influence; rather it is that although a necessary, it is not a sufficient condition to change clinical policy.

Therefore, the promotion of clinical policy change, whether in response to medical practice variations or to other imperatives, seems possible through two general strategies. In the one case the medical profession must recognise the less than scientific influences on medical practice, and adopt strategies that will use these influences to develop scientific evidence into clinical policy, i.e. moving away from the historic reliance on traditional educational routes. Not only must they predispose towards change by establishing national guidelines for practice which are well grounded in the scientific literature – which they are starting to do – but also they must take responsibility for creative local initiatives to enable and reinforce adherence to the standard. The reasons for resistance to such a strategy, and a case study of one such approach, are presented in the next section.

The attraction of this strategy to the medical profession should be its ability, if enacted responsibly, to retain for themselves the decisions over what constitutes appropriate practice and how it will be implemented – the maintenance of clinical freedom. The alternative will capitalise on the observation that the influences at the local level can be bypassed, or overwhelmed, by direct economic or administrative regulation of inappropriate practice. This second general strategy will involve standards imposed from without by government or other third party payers, and, while physicians will probably not be predisposed towards policy change, such change will nevertheless be forcefully enabled and reinforced by economic incentives. The clinical freedom of the profession will be secondary to their economic bondage. The mechanics and the problems of this alternative are addressed in the final section.

PROMOTING CHANGE FROM WITHIN THE MEDICAL PROFESSION

The above discussion of influences on clinical policy has abstracted from the impact of the specific presenting symptoms and signs of individual patients. It is assumed that a major influence on the specific decisions regarding a specific patient will be the perceived benefit that will accrue from applying a clinical policy in this particular case. However, the important word here is the *perceived* benefit. The inherent uncertainties in medical decision making leave plenty of room for the myriad of non-scientific influences to edge out what actually is best for the patient, replacing it with a less scientifically justifiable course of action, but still leaving a genuinely held perception of benefit (Eddy, 1984). Inappropriate clinical policies are not maliciously or manipulatively maintained.

However, although this focus of the physician on the individual patient encounter is an important strategy for dealing with the uncertainty, it is also misleading. When the 'unit of analysis' is each individual patient, the perceptions of benefit typically become biased. For instance, the impact of the last case on the management of the current patient (especially if it was a particularly adverse or positive outcome) is out of all proportion to the scientific weight that should be attached to one patient among many. Therefore, a more dispassionate source of influence is required. It is for this purpose that the scientific research evidence exists and, more recently, 'official policies' summarising this evidence are being produced by national specialty societies or task forces (Fowkes and Roberts, 1984).

To the extent that the medical profession is increasingly engaging in exercises to set 'official clinical policy', then they are starting to address the challenge of medical practice variation and the changing of inappropriate 'individual clinical policy'.* The medical profession is the obvious candidate to produce such official policy, because it has the detailed knowledge that gives the competitive edge over non-physicians to appraise and promulgate the research evidence. The credibility of such policies is also immeasurably enhanced when they are the product of forces from within, rather than from outside, the medical profession. Therefore, once the need for policy change has been identified, the medical profession, as a corporate body and not as individuals, should be the agent of first choice.

However, the distance of this policy setting from the local environment, as discussed above, casts it at best in the role of predisposing towards, but not enabling or reinforcing, change. Unfortunately, there is significant resistance at the local level even to these distant official policies. To receive acceptance they must be sold as guidelines and not standards for practice, otherwise they are perceived as a threat to the individual autonomy of practitioners and their right to discretion at the level of each patient encounter. Therefore, strategies to enact these official policies must take place at the local level, both because this increases the probability that they will respect the desire of physicians at

---

*There is an ethical issue buried in this increasing trend towards setting official clinical policies. If it is thought that the policy might have any influence on the actual behaviour of practitioners, they should take great care to reflect a dispassionate appraisal of the scientific evidence and avoid the substitution of personal opinion. There must be assurance that there is an extremely low probability of the suggested policy doing more harm than the current practice pattern. Thus, techniques for setting such official policies should reflect our knowledge of how to ensure that the final product is largely based on evidence, not personal predilection (Lomas et al., 1988).

least to feel as if they have maintained signficant discretion over patient management, and because it is at the local level that enabling and reinforcing influences for change are found.

In the context of rising to the challenge of medical practice variations, the stages in the strategy are triggered by the demonstration of variation. The first stage is to promulgate and disseminate the official clinical policy at the national level, i.e. predispose towards change in the area of practice where variations have demonstrated an uncertainty as to the appropriate clinical policy. The second stage is to facilitate the policy's incorporation into local practice environments by exploiting enough of the non-scientific influences on decision making for actual behaviour change towards the policy to be enabled and reinforced. There is a touch of Machiavelli in this process, because the underlying philosophy is that one cares not *why* the policy change occurs, only that it does occur. In an ideal world we would wish that these behaviour changes would occur solely because of exposure to, and education from, scientific information. In reality, however, the behaviour change will occur through peer pressure, marketing of information and exploitation of informal communication channels. This tactic was learnt long ago by the pharmaceutical companies. Their national targeted advertising predisposes towards change in prescribing behaviour, but it is the visits from the local drug company representative and the local presentations from credible and respected peers that actually enables the change to occur (Avorn *et al.*, 1982).

A CASE STUDY

Since 1984 a group of us in Canada have been applying the principles of this strategy to achieve clinical policy change in one area of obstetrical practice – the use of caesarean section. We first demonstrated practice variation and identified the areas that were of greatest concern (Anderson and Lomas, 1984, 1985). This information was used to gain the co-operation and endorsement of the national obstetrical society, which engaged in a consensus development exercise to generate an 'official policy' for the use of caesarean section (Panel of the National Consensus Conference on Aspects of Cesarean Birth, 1986). This consensus statement was disseminated to every practising obstetrician in Canada. Our evaluation, using self-report surveys, indicates that 1 year after release in excess of 90% of obstetricians were aware of its existence and 85% agreed with its recommendations. Two years after its release 34% of obstetricians and 33% of hospitals claimed that they had changed their clinical policies on the basis of the statement.

Unfortunately, hospitals and obstetricians appear to confuse predis-position towards change with actual change. Hospital discharge data for the 2 years following release of the statement indicate little or no significant change. In Figures 10.1 and 10.2 the data are presented from Canada's largest province for the overall caesarean section rate and the rate for one of the most important indications – previous caesarean section – for the 4 years prior to, and the 2 years following, release of the statement. The arrow on each figure indicates the release of the statement. If the recommendations of the official policy had been followed, both of these rates would have dropped significantly. The data indicate that at best the national dissemination of the official policy halted an ongoing increase in these rates, but it certainly did not result in full compliance with, or a change of policy in accordance with, the recommendations of the statement. This finding replicates other nega-tive outcomes from evaluations of the impact of national consensus statements on practice behaviour (Kosecoff *et al.*, 1987; Hill *et al.*, 1988).

These results were no surprise to us, given the evidence that national policy achieves no more than predisposition towards clinical policy change. The application of our second stage – exploitation of local influences on practice to enable and reinforce change – is currently under way. Initially it involved an extensive literature review to find proven effective strategies for changing clinical policy at the local level (Lomas and Haynes, 1988). One of our criteria for the selection of strategies was that they could be used by the medical profession itself if

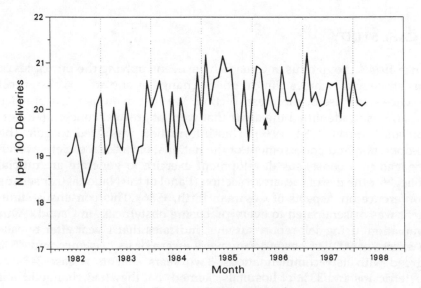

Figure 10.1 Caesarean section rates, by month

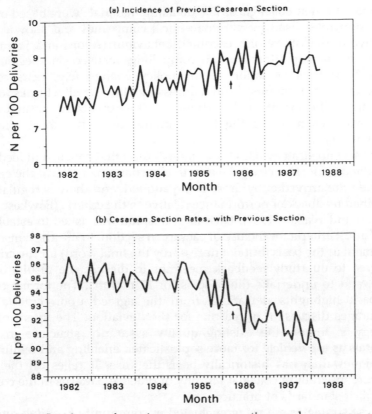

Figure 10.2 Incidence of previous caesarean section, and caesarean section rates with previous section, by month

they proved to be effective in the context of changing inappropriate clinical policies.

Two strategies have been selected (Lomas, 1988).

First, educationally influential local physicians were identified by a technique based on sociograms (Stross and Bole, 1980). Physicians with obstetrical privileges at the local hospital were asked by mail to volunteer the names of colleagues who best matched brief descriptions of archetypal concerned and informed physicians. The most frequently mentioned individual was designated as the 'educational influential' in the community. These physicians were then brought to a workshop and educated on the background evidence in support of the consensus statement, and have now been sent back into the community with a request to maintain their usual network of contacts and encourage implementation of the statement. These physicians were also given 'detailing materials' based on different aspects of the statement to distribute to their colleagues. The detailing materials were based on the same principles used by pharmaceutical companies and shown to be effective in one study of prescribing behaviour (Avorn and Soumerai, 1983), i.e. visually attractive and compelling, focused on specific concerns over implementation of the policy change (e.g. fears of the malpractice implications), and addressing 'bite-sized' chunks of information. The intent of this strategy is to exploit the natural communication channels of the local community in the most effective possible way.

The second strategy uses the demonstration that concurrent feedback of audited performance can be effective in changing policy if the criteria for audit are arrived at by those being audited, and there is regular and sustained feedback of performance relative to the criteria (Fowkes, 1982; Haynes and Walker, 1987). Each local hospital was asked to establish a set of audit criteria for the use of caesarean section, to use the consensus statement as the basis (but not necessarily the final word) for the criteria, to agree to quarterly feedback meetings to discuss the results of the audit, and to undertake the process for 12 months. The format of the feedback highlights deviations from the agreed upon criteria and encourages discussion of reasons for the deviation. The intent of this strategy is to use the existing quality assurance structure in local hospitals as the vehicle for more sophisticated enabling and reinforcing techniques than has historically been the case. It relies on the peer pressure inherent in collegial scrutiny of practice patterns in the context of explicit standards of practice.

These strategies are being evaluated in community hospitals and are being compared in a randomised trial format with a baseline condition in which local obstetricians merely receive a repeat mailing of the published consensus statement. The 'intervention period' is not yet complete; therefore, outcomes for the two strategies, which have been shown effective in other contexts, are not yet available.

THE CHALLENGE FOR THE MEDICAL PROFESSION

The above study is being conducted in a 'research and development' context such that the results can be immediately adopted by specialty societies, medical associations, licensing bodies, medical advisory committees of hospitals and other medical organisations in a programme format.

For instance, if the local educational influential (EI) proves to be an effective enabling and reinforcing agent for policy change, specialty societies can identify their EI in each community and use them as the conduit to all local physicians for the communication of official clinical policies, relevant research findings or concerns about practice variations. If the audit and concurrent feedback strategy is effective, then a national organisation to facilitate such activity could be funded by the medical profession, and mandated to assist local communities to use their existing quality assurance structures in this proven effective fashion. This is not dissimilar to the model already adopted in Holland by the CBO – an organisation that is also responsible for the production of predisposing national consensus statements to use in the enabling and reinforcing process of hospital-based audit (Casparie *et al.*, 1987).

These strategies impose an expectation on the medical profession to take substantive and not just symbolic action to change clinical policies in the face of medical practice variations. The promulgation of practice standards at a remote national level is little more than a symbolic attack on the problem. It does satisfy the need, internal to the profession, to avoid encroachment on individuals' clinical discretion and autonomy while, for the present, giving a public appearance of doing something. However, it will not be long before it becomes widely known that standards set from afar, and labelled only as guidelines, are changing little out in the field of medical practice. It is when this realisation dawns on the consumers and payers for medical care that the profession will have to make the choice between maintaining control over clinical policy change within the profession by adopting new strategies – for instance, ones similar to those outlined above – or standing by as forces from outside the profession impose clinical policy change, using the economic incentive tools at their disposal. Clinical policy change in response to medical practice variations *can* be achieved from within the medical profession, but it will require the profession to confront the 'art' in medicine and to exploit those non-scientific influences on practice in ways that may threaten some of the current tenets of discretion, individual autonomy and individual (rather than professional) clinical freedom.

REGULATING CHANGE FROM WITHOUT

Public policy for medical care has always been a walk on a tightrope between respect for the right of physicians to practice medicine as they see fit and respect for the right of taxpayers to hold government accountable for its expenditures. Until recently, this balancing act clearly favoured the profession's right over the content of medical practice. Demonstrations of medical practice variations, among other things, are starting to alter that balance. For the first time those who fund medical care are asking questions about what they are funding. But asking questions is still a long way from directly regulating clinical policy.

To hold the right over medical practice to be sacrosanct imposes certain public policy imperatives upon those who fund care. Foremost among these imperatives is the need, once a problem has been identified in medical practice, to afford the medical profession a chance to put their own house in order. Medical practice variations have now been identified as a problem and those who fund care are waiting for the house to be put in order. Whether the period of grace allowed the medical profession will be short or long will depend on the effectiveness of the profession's symbolic responses and on the degree to which fiscal imperatives intrude. But eventually the absence of a substantive response from the profession will bring a substitute response from those who fund care.

The beginnings of this approach can be seen in the USA, where the significant private sector presence in health care funding means that much of the management of the health care system is not directly encumbered by the political constraints of government. Faced with medical practice variations, their response has been to establish and impose, through independent utilisation review organisations, their own standards of allowable care. The strategy has been to use the administrative and economic influences on clinical policy outlined earlier. Thus, the US physician is becoming accustomed to practising in hospitals with a metaphorical monkey on one shoulder, second-guessing and questioning every clinical decision, and an accountant on the other shoulder, advising and informing on the current allowable billing practices.

Unfortunately, the motivating factor behind this strategy to change clinical policy is principally financial and only secondarily the quality of care. The goals of these agents of change from outside the medical profession would be achieved if all areas were reduced to the same level of intervention as the lowest rates found across different regions. Medical practice variations are a signal for them that the lowest rates will do. Evidence from the USA does give some cause for concern that this imposition of relatively uninformed clinical policy change from outside is less preferable to a more informed change process from within the profession itself. For instance, Chassin and colleagues have found, in a study of practice variations in the treatment of the elderly in the USA, that the areas with the lowest rates had equivalent proportions of inappropriate care to those of areas with the highest rates (Chassin *et al.*, 1986). Thus, reducing all areas to the same level of intervention as the lowest rate will do little to improve the appropriateness of care. Furthermore, although it has been shown that private utilisation review programmes do contain costs (Feldstein *et al.*, 1988), there are some suggestions that hospitals operating in such regulated environments have higher inpatient mortality rates than those outside this influence (Shortell and Hughes, 1988).

These results merely underline why the medical profession is the preferred agent to achieve change in clinical policy – they potentially have the expertise and the motivation to tie the policy change to health outcomes rather than just cost outcomes.

But governments need not pursue the same policies as the US private sector if the medical profession fails to respond. The additional public accountability of governments as medical care funding agents will probably lead to a more sophisticated marshalling of the influences on clinical policy in a way that takes greater account of quality of care as well as expenditure levels. For instance, in those countries where fee schedules are the principal form of reimbursement, there is no reason why the relative values of fees cannot be calibrated to promote appropriate clinical policies established by the profession's guidelines or standards of practice. Once the medical profession's failure to respond justifies this outside intrusion on clinical freedom, the many influences comprising the art of medicine open up numerous channels through which the science of medicine can be creatively injected into clinical policies by governments or their agents. Exit physicians, chased by Machiavellian outsiders.

ACKNOWLEDGEMENTS

The author receives personal support as a Career Scientist from the Ontario Ministry of Health. Much of the work reported in this chapter was supported by a grant from the National Health Research and Development Programme, Health and Welfare, Canada.

REFERENCES

Anderson, G. M. and Lomas, J. (1984). Determinants of the increasing cesarean birth rate: Ontario data 1979 to 1982. *New England Journal of Medicine*, **311**, 887–92

Anderson, G. M. and Lomas, J. (1985). Explaining variations in cesarean section rates: Patients, facilities or policies? *Canadian Medical Association Journal*, **132**, 253–9

Avorn, J., Chen, M. and Hartley, R. (1982). Scientific versus commercial sources of influence on the prescribing behaviour of physicians. *American Journal of Medicine*, **73**, 4–8

Avorn, J. and Soumerai, S. B. (1983). Improving drug-therapy decisions through educational outreach. A randomized trial of academically based 'detailing'. *New England Journal of Medicine*, **308**, 1457–63

Barer, M. L., Evans, R. G. and Labelle, R. J. (1988). Fee controls as cost control: Tales from the frozen north. *Milbank Quarterly*, **66**, 1–64

Brook, R. H., Park, R. E., Winslow, C. M., Kosecoff, J. B., Chassin, M. R. and Hampton, J. R. (1988). Diagnosis and treatment of coronary disease: Comparison of doctors' attitudes in the USA and the UK. *Lancet*, 2 April, 750–3

Casparie, A. F., Klazinga, N. S., Everdingen, J. J. and Touw, P. P. (1987). Health care providers resolve clinical controversies: The Dutch consensus approach. *Australian Clinical Review*, March, 43–7

Chassin, M. R., Brook, R. H., Park, R. E. *et al.* (1986). Variations in the use of medical and surgical services by the Medicare population. *New England Journal of Medicine*, **314**, 285–90

Eddy, D. M. (1982). Clinical policies and the quality of clinical practice. *New England Journal of Medicine*, **307**, 343–7

Eddy, D. M. (1984). Variations in physician practice: the role of uncertainty. *Health Affairs*, **3**, 74–89

Eisenberg, J. M. (1985). Physician utilization: The state of research about physicians' practice patterns. *Medical Care*, **23**, 461–83

Eisenberg, J. M. (1986). *Doctors' Decisions and the Cost of Medical Care*. Health Administration Press, Ann Arbor, Michigan

Evans, C. E., Haynes, R. B. and Birkett, N. J. (1986). Does a mailed continuing education program improve physician performance? Results of a randomized trial in antihypertensive care. *Journal of the American Medical Association*, **255**, 501–4

Feldstein, P. J., Wickizer, T. M. and Wheeler, J. R. (1988). Private cost containment: the effects of utilization review programs on health care use and expenditures. *New England Journal of Medicine*, **318**, 1310–14

Fowkes, F. G. (1982). Medical audit cycle: a review of methods and research in clinical practice. *Medical Education*, **16**, 228–38

Fowkes, F. G. and Roberts, C. J. (1984). Introducing guidelines into clinical practice. *Effective Health Care*, **1**, 313–23

Green, L. W. and Eriksen, M. P. (1988). Behavioural determinants of preventive practices by physicians. *American Journal of Preventive Medicine*, **4**(Suppl.), 101–7

Greer, A. L. (1987). The two cultures of biomedicine: can there be consensus? *Journal of the American Medical Association*, **258**, 2739–40

Greer, A. L. (1988). The state of the art versus the state of the science: the diffusion of new medical technologies into practice. *International Journal of Technology Assessment in Health Care*, **4**, 5–26

Haynes, R. B., Davis, D. A., McKibbon, K. A. and Tugwell, P. (1984). A critical appraisal of the efficacy of continuing medical education. *Journal of the American Medical Association*, **251**, 61–4

Haynes, R. B. and Walker, C. J. (1987). Computer-aided quality assurance: a critical appraisal. *Archives of Internal Medicine*, **147**, 1297–1304

Hill, M. N., Levine, D. M. and Whelton, P. K. (1988). Awareness, use, and impact of the 1984 Joint National Committee Consensus Report on high blood pressure. *American Journal of Public Health*, **78**, 1190–4

Jacoby, I. and Clark, S. A. (1986). Direct mailing as a means of disseminating NIH consensus statements: a comparison with current techniques. *Journal of the American Medical Association*, **255**, 1328–30

Kosecoff, J., Kanouse, D. E., Rogers, W. H. *et al.*.(1987). Effects of the National Institutes of Health Consensus Development Programme on physician practice. *Journal of the American Medical Association*, **258**, 2708–13

Lomas, J. (1988). Holding back the tide of caesareans: publishing recommendations is not enough to stop the rise. *British Medical Journal*, **297**, 569–70

Lomas, J., Anderson, G. M., Enkin, M., Vayda, E., Roberts, R. and MacKinnon, B. A. (1988). The role of evidence in the consensus process: results from a Canadian consensus exercise. *Journal of the American Medical Association*, **259**, 3001–5

Lomas, J. and Haynes, R. B. (1988). A taxonomy and critical review of tested strategies for the application of clinical practice recommendations: from 'official' to 'individual' clinical policy. *American Journal of Preventive Medicine*, **4**(Suppl.), 78–93

McClure, W. (1982). Toward development and application of a qualitative theory of hospital utilization. *Inquiry*, **19**, 117–35

Panel of the National Consensus Conference on Aspects of Cesarean Birth (1986). Final statement of The Panel of the National Consensus Conference on Aspects of Cesarean Birth. *Canadian Medical Association Journal*, **134**, 1348–52

Retchin, S. M., Fletcher, R. H., Buescher, P. C. *et al.* (1985). The application of official policy: prophylaxis recommendations for patients with mitral valve prolapse. *Medical Care*, **23**, 1156–62

Schroeder, S. A. (1987). Strategies for reducing medical costs by changing physicians' behaviour: efficacy and impact on quality of care. *International Journal of Technology Assessment in Health Care*, **3**, 39–50

Schroeder, S. A., Myers, L. P. and McPhee, S. J. (1984). The failure of physician education as a cost-containment strategy: report of the prospective controlled trial at a university hospital. *Journal of the American Medical Association*, **252**, 225–30

Shortell, S. M. and Hughes, E. F. (1988). The effects of regulation, competition, and ownership on mortality rates among hospital inpatients. *New England Journal of Medicine*, **318**, 1100–7

Stross, J. K. and Bole, G. G. (1980). Evaluation of a continuing education program in rheumatoid arthritis. *Arthritis and Rheumatism*, **23**, 846–9

Vayda, E. (1973). A comparison of surgical rates in Canada and in England and Wales. *New England Journal of Medicine*, **289**, 1224–9

Wennberg, J. E., Blowers, L., Parker, R. and Gittelsohn, A. M. (1977). Changes in tonsillectomy rates associated with feedback and review. *Pediatrics*, **59**, 821–6

Winkler, J. D., Lohr, K. N. and Brook, R. H. (1985). Persuasive communication and medical technology assessment. *Archives of Internal Medicine*, **145**, 314–17

CHAPTER 11

Challenges Facing Modern Health Care

Gavin Mooney and Tavs Folmer Andersen

A NEED FOR CHANGE

The evidence on medical practice variations in this book, and the discussions of various facets and implications of these, point in our view to at least one very clear, unambiguous conclusion. Whatever best medical practice is, however 'doing one's best for one's patients' is construed, not all doctors are doing it. That basic point is central to all that has gone before in this book. It is fundamental to the challenges facing health care and the medical profession in the years ahead.

The mere existence of medical practice variation has been a well-known and implicitly accepted aspect of health care for a long time. But what really constitutes a new situation is the overwhelming amount of evidence which is now becoming available. There is no longer a black box in which medicine may be practised. In the age of information technology, patterns of medical practice will be a public issue. Everybody, including the medical profession, health care administrators, health policy makers, actual and potential patients, will have to acknowledge the existence of gross variations in medical practice. Such variations seem to prevail in a large proportion of all activities of modern health services, and it is becoming rather obvious that the basis for decision making at the clinical level, as well as at the administrative and policy making level, is inadequate.

Fundamental problems need to be clarified to improve the current situation and to reduce inappropriate variation in medical practice (see McPherson, in this volume). At the very basic level, there is a need to clarify the goals and objectives of health services to be provided by each health care system, according to its cultural, ethical and political setting. For example, the weight that different societies attach to equity, an important consideration with regard to variations, tends to differ from one to another (see Bevan, in this volume). As the emphasis of care is gradually shifting away from mere prolongation of life towards improvement of the quality of life, this need becomes more and more urgent to allow priority setting in health care. Secondly, a substantial need for better information on the effectiveness and efficiency of available technologies has been identified as a key problem. Many new technologies have been introduced and widely disseminated through our health services, without ever being sufficiently evaluated, and in the current situation it is virtually impossible to navigate our health services on the basis of rational decision making.

In recent years there has been concern in various quarters at the increasing cost of health care and a view that there was a need for 'cost containment' to stop 'cost escalation'. This has, perhaps inevitably, led to some concern among the medical profession, particularly with respect to a potential threat to their autonomy. And given the health concerns of the population and the way in which health care is (at least) subsidised and often zero-priced at the point of consumption, it is perhaps only natural that the public have sided with the doctors. It is easy to work up an emotional case for what Fuchs has called the 'romantic' cause in health care, i.e. attempting to ignore the fact that resources are limited (Fuchs, 1974). Faced with the 'white coats and stethoscopes' arguments and the prognoses of the economists, the white coats will tend to win.

Historically, societies have delegated a lot of responsibility to the medical profession and, consequently, the anatomy of modern health services has been developed primarily by well-established medical decision makers. The potential consequences of this reliance on ato-mised decisions, being made in every medical specialty, are exemplified by the so-called 'surgical signatures'. What might appear to be rational decisions, when seen in their own local context of the specialties, may result in capriciousness at the level of the total health services. The more or less haphazard mix of health care activities utilised by populations, which are otherwise apparently similar, should thus be interpreted as a warning: the clinical decision forum of the past and present is not an appropriate place to settle important priorities in health care.

But the monopoly on information about what those inside the white coats were doing to their patients is now broken, or, perhaps more accurately, there has been an intrusion into the ignorance of what they have been doing (see Wennberg, in this volume). It is now not so clear that the romantic will side with the doctor or perhaps he or she will change from being a romantic. Medical practice variations indicate to all those who are prepared to take notice of them that given the right to do what he or she thinks is best for his or her patients, a doctor does just that – maybe. But strictly we do not know this from the evidence. Doctors do different things. Is this because their bests are different? Or are some of them not achieving their bests?

It is not intended to imply that individual doctors are to blame for the extent of variations in the sense of laying fault at their doors. The fact that they do different things is at least in part a function of the fact that societies let them do different things. The medical profession is normally to a very considerable extent left to regulate itself. The rest of us do not know enough about what constitutes medicine, and certainly not about what constitutes the technical aspects of good practice, to be responsible for such a regulation. Much better, has been the view, to let the professional experts regulate the profession. Self-regulation is presumed to be the answer.

Or perhaps with the better data sources now available (see Roos *et al.*, in this volume) and with the widening knowledge we have of the existence of medical practice variations, it might be more accurate to say: 'self-regulation was thought to be the answer'. Where both self-interest and society's interests are at stake, it is always potentially dangerous to leave matters to the self-interested, no matter how great their social concerns. Yet societies have felt able to do so in the case of the medical profession. Medical practice variation represents an important challenge to that view and a potential challenge to the profession, as Vestergaard, from a lay perspective, brings out in this volume. Can they put their own house in order? A prior question: are they willing to recognise medical practice variation as a sympton of a potentially serious ailment in the corporate medical body (see Lomas, in this volume)? Perhaps we have reached the point, where traditional medical, self-regulation of health care must give way to other types of regulation, based on aggregate societal, rather than partial professional rationality.

Objectives of Change

Something is wrong. Can and will the profession sort it out? A number of strategies are possible here. At one extreme is the view that merely by illuminating the evidence of medical practice variation, the profession will see the error of their ways and attempt to rectify the problem. Such a view assumes that the profession accepts 'getting it right' as a principle which overrides all other considerations. That, in its extreme form at least, seems most unlikely. Doctors do have interests beyond those of their patients. But it also assumes that somebody somewhere, knows what 'getting it right' means. One of the great difficulties about the evidence to date on change as a result of the presentation of evidence on variations to the professionals involved is that, since no one seems to know what is optimal, it is difficult to form a judgement on whether any change is better or worse. One can put forward reasonable arguments that more informed choice is better, but the philosophy of 'cosiness' – all getting together around some common mean or standard and not being an antisocial outlier – can only be seen as virtuous if the point on the scale around which cosiness occurs is based on some rationale.

The challenge here is not variation *per se*: it is trying to discover where cosiness should occur, and the extent to which it is a virtue (see Mulley, in this volume). Some forms of variation are more acceptable than others.

However, it is important to note that even in small countries and states, where practising physicians tend to know each other very well, it is often a surprising experience for them to be confronted with the evidence of the multitude of practice styles as, for instance, represented in population-based rates of well-known interventions. Being faced with this reality, it becomes demanding to distinguish those areas, where cosiness of professional consensus may be enjoyed from other areas, where true disagreement and professional uncertainty prevail. This is where practice variation becomes pregnant and begins to point in the direction of 'organised medicine' at a higher level.

At the other extreme, it can be argued that, since there is substantial evidence of variation but little evidence of substance that higher activity levels are better than lower activity levels, at least lower activity costs less, and that, *ceteris paribus*, is a virtue. Cost containment is then the *ceteris paribus*er's goal.

But is the *ceretis paribus* assumption justified? It might be; indeed, it may well be. What is needed is evidence, not of variation *per se* but of what variations mean in terms of both relevant outputs (primarily health) and resource use. There is a very serious lack here, and an important challenge lies not only in much better and much more extensive measurement of effectiveness, but also in much more concern with thinking about effectiveness of resource use, i.e efficiency. The profession has for too long attempted to fulfil the requirements for Victor Fuchs' romanticism. The challenge is for the profession to accept that efficiency matters and that they, both as a corporate medical profession and as individual practitioners, have a role to play in pursuing it both in getting to grips with measuring effectiveness and in taking more responsibility for the deployment of society's scarce resources.

However, it must be kept in mind that for many common interventions there is currently no way to determine an 'appropriate level of utilisation', partly because the evidence on effectiveness is not sufficient, and partly because there is no consensus on what 'appropriate' means in this context. While 'small may be beautiful' in the context of cost containment, a simple-minded strategy based on the outlawing of high utilisation areas could run the risk of containing health and quality of life as well. On the other hand, if high-rate areas are being 'overserviced', a reduction would lead to improved efficiency, the 'medicalised' population would escape 'unnecessary' treatment, and they (and perhaps others) unnecessary costs.

For decision makers and policy makers in health care, the difficult task of allocating resources is like navigating a ship in foggy weather close to the magnetic North Pole, where even the compass does not know where to go for the true North.

However, it is up to the medical profession to prove that the cost containers' *ceteris paribus* assumption is wrong. The onus is on the profession to do so, although certainly they need to accept the role of other health disciplines in addressing the issue.

Between the 'let's leave it to the profession to put its house in order' extreme and the 'high is bad, *ceteris paribus*, because it's costly' extreme there are many possible positions to adopt. Our view is that the solution does lie in between. And it lies very simply – in principle at least – in accepting the goal of efficiency, which involves taking account of both effectiveness and resource use. Best medical practice is efficient medical practice. (It is worth noting that that does not mean necessarily that efficient medical practice lies somwhere in between the current highs and lows. We don't even know that!)

To aim at efficiency as the goal for good medical care has important consequences for the traditional monopoly position of the medical profession. It has become obvious that the 'partial rationality' of specialised medicine has not so far been, and will not in future be, able to attain the goal without involving a broad range of disciplines in health sciences, and without involving the politics of priority setting.

Knowledge for Change

While the medical profession and the policy makers are immediately confronted with the challenges of medical practice variations, substantial responsibilites are also emerging for the international research community in health services. As indicated in the previous chapters, a very substantial amount of research is called for in a number of disciplines. However, the real challenge of the coming age will be to develop an integrated, coherent evaluative science as a basis for decision making at all levels of our health services.

This development is currently at an early stage, and much attention must be devoted to interdisciplinary as well as international collaboration before the necessary new paradigms can be developed. One of the important regions of interdisciplinary growth and future proliferation has been mapped through the previous chapters, involving a number of relatively autonomous disciplines in health services research such as statistics, epidemiology, sociology, economics and decision analysis.

The need for cross-fertilisation between such research disciplines is especially urgent, given our current lack of knowledge with regard to causes and consequences of practice variation. To fill in this gap is going to require a very substantial investment in a co-ordinated strategy for health services research over the coming years (see Wennberg, in this volume).

Studies of variation in utilisation and outcomes of medical care have grown out of a multitude of disciplines, including epidemiology, statistics, clinical and social sciences. Major methodological advances have already been made, but there is still a long way to go before the causes and consequences of practice variation will be understood fully. It is *here* that increased priority is needed and not just a description, as in the past.

The amount of evidence of practice variation has grown immensely over the last 15 years. However, it must be appreciated that for each and every health care system the phenomenon presents itself in a unique context. Consequently, more studies of utilisation patterns are needed to allow proper standards for clinical decision making and policy prescriptions to be worked out at the detailed level. However, the evidence of the existence of variations is there in more than adequate amount for policy makers to be concerned.

Given the societal acceptance of many common health care interventions which have never been subject to sufficient evaluation, particularly with respect to effectiveness and efficiency, it is crucial to develop further strategies for non-experimental research. Unfortunately, many of the most important questions in current medical practice cannot be addressed through powerful experimental methodologies, such as have been required for a long time in drug therapy. The real challenge, then, is to accept the necessity of relying on evidence produced in the 'natural setting', where patients are being referred and selected for treatment according to highly variable standards. Even though this may seem to be close to impossible, recent developments of methodologies in outcomes research show that powerful tools are available (see Roos *et al.*, in this volume).

While the study of variation in utilisation and outcomes of medical care – to some extent – has been established as a scientific field within health services research, there is a need to link up with other related areas, such as medical decision analysis and health economics – especially as it is in these areas that the scope for *explaining* variations is greatest.

The medical decision-making models that exist can be, but seldom are, adapted for helping to explain medical practice variation. However, decision analysis provides a valuable tool to summarise and evaluate the implications of existing, or even hypothetical knowledge concerning effectiveness of alternative available treatments (see Mulley, in this volume).

The goal of medical practice is often constrained too narrowly but ought to reflect better, and indeed more often try to find out, what the relevant maximand is, rather than assuming it. Medical decision analysis is a potentially very fruitful source for explaining variation and it is in the better explanation of variations that future research has to concentrate to allow future policy tools to be suitably honed and efficiently directed. Indeed, a key challenge here lies in greater linking of the objectives of medical practice with the objectives of health care. Do doctors do different things under different financing arrangements? Does this matter? Are there better/worse ways of financing health care to pursue best medical practice? What constitutes 'legitimate' variation? How autonomous can the individual patient be? should he/she be? How can we allow for (should we allow for?) variations in the personality of the doctor – for example, with respect to attitudes to risk?

The research on medical decision making needs to be used in the future in at least three distinct ways: first, helping to provide better explanations of variations; second, sorting out the 'legitimate' from the 'illegitimate' component of variation; and third, identifying the key uncertainties in the existing assessment of effectiveness. Realising this potential of medical decision analysis is one of the key research challenges for the future.

With some honourable exceptions, health economists have tended to ignore the phenomenon of medical practice variation, beyond their considerable concern about and with supplier-induced demand. Clearly, this is an important source of variation, but, perhaps because of the emphasis placed on it, economists have tended to contribute little else to the debate on variations. And with their (at least in the eyes of the medical profession) close association with the cost containers their voice has had little impact on the issue of best medical practice.

Economists need more often to link with the variations researchers and the medical decision analysts to help first to conceptualise best medical practice and second to put empirical flesh on the conceptual bones so that (efficient) standards of practice can be established. It is not suggested that these will be tablets of stone. They are likely to vary from country to country for various reasons, but particularly because of different levels of resource availability and of different valuations of health and thereby priorities. They are also likely to vary within countries at least partially for the same reasons. The key here is in demonstrating how to set efficient standards in practice – and indeed how not to! (See McGuire, in this volume.)

However, where the economist community has to do more is in identifying those forms of primarily medical but also patient behaviour most conducive to the promotion of best medical practice. Beyond that the economists need also to identify those financing, budgeting and remuneration arrangements most likely to create the right incentives to ensure that efficiency is pursued (see Evans, in this volume).

However, where the key lies for research at least – but it quickly moves into policy concerns – is in these three bodies of researchers – the epidemiologists, the decision analysts and the economists – getting co-operatively to grips with what is fundamental to all other considerations: the identification of the objectives and values of, first, health care systems and, second (but of course linked), medical decision making. In this regard, each health care system, embedded in its own specific cultural identity, may well differ. However, to allow proper conceptualisation, planning and evaluation of the performance of the system, such objectives and values need to be made explicit. Advances in health care technology are large and growing in number. Many make small, even insignificant advances to health, even if they advance health care expenditure. This emphasises the need to clarify objectives and values, to evaluate and to do so *ex ante* and not just *ex post*. With accelerating innovative changes in medical technology, it is likely that before one wakes up each morning, yet another new horse has been put between the shafts. But before having to buy and feed the new horses, we would like to know whether they are any better than the old ones. We should also make up our minds as to which cargo the horses are supposed to be pulling, and in which direction. Clinicians do not exchange their kingdoms for their technological horses. Medical innovations too often serve as a means of furthering imperial ambitions without sufficient consideration of effectiveness and efficiency.

CHALLENGES OF MEDICAL PRACTICE VARIATION

Variation is an intrinsic and fertile aspect of human life. It can be a source of inspiration and growth. Medical practice variation is no exception, in so far as the phenomenon is a reflection of reasonably rational mechanisms in the delivery of health care. However, the accumulated evidence on practice variation indicates patterns of utilisation which are in sharp contrast to the prevailing myths regarding the basis of modern health care delivery.

While practice variation is by no means an exclusively modern phenomenon, the apparent heterogeneity of modern medical care is counter-indicative of the very popular view that medical practice is based on a coherent body of scientific knowledge. Maybe the most important virtue of the results of practice variation studies is the implication that apparently similar populations are exposed to grossly different patterns of care, both from a quantitative and from a qualitative point of view. If this could all be 'scientifically' justified, maybe we need a better science – and so we do.

The appreciation of dramatic regional differences in the composition of health care activities involves important questions about the health of populations and the utilisation of resources. As a consequence of its historical role, the medical profession has had the privilege to influence greatly the development of our modern health care systems. However, the apparent inadequacies in the ability of modern health care systems to optimise efficient and equitable utilisation of care indicates a need for shared responsibility, with input from many disciplines.

As the level and growth of health care expenditures have become a real concern in countries with highly developed health care systems, the evidence on practice variation provides good ammunition for the battle of explicit priority setting in modern health care. Whatever the current implicit goals of activities in health care may be, it is obvious from variation research that priorities are already being set, but according to varying principles. The necessary health policy battle, then, will require a threefold process of: first, making the current goals explicit; second, working towards a consensus, which is strong enough for the purpose of policy making and priority setting; and third, providing the right sets of incentives to get the various actors in the system to pursue health service goals efficiently.

In conclusion, medical practice variation represents a great challenge to modern health care. While *some* variation must be considered as a justified and legitimate aspect of all human activities, there is enough evidence to indicate that medical practice varies well beyond such limits.

We are faced with differences which should be regarded as evidence that there are very definite problems in decision making at all levels of health care. What we need is a three fold clarification: to clarify the goals of health care; to come up with the means to reach these goals; *and* how to get people motivated to achieve the goals. Even if the causes of practice variation are far from being understood in every detail, the evidence is there for posing very important questions. We have to find the answers.

REFERENCE

Fuchs, V. R. (1974). *Who Shall Live? Health, Economics, and Social Choice.* Basic Books, New York

Index